Regression Analysis of Survival Data in Cancer Chemotherapy

STATISTICS: Textbooks and Monographs

A SERIES EDITED BY

D. B. OWEN, Coordinating Editor
Department of Statistics
Southern Methodist University
Dallas, Texas

R. G. CORNELL, Associate Editor for Biostatistics
School of Public Health
University of Michigan
Ann Arbor, Michigan

OTHER VOLUMES IN PREPARATION

Regression Analysis of Survival Data in Cancer Chemotherapy

WALTER H. CARTER, Jr.

Departments of Biostatistics and Medicine
Medical College of Virginia
Virginia Commonwealth University
Richmond, Virginia

GALEN L. WAMPLER

Department of Medicine
Medical College of Virginia
Richmond, Virginia

DONALD M. STABLEIN

The Emmes Corporation
Potomac, Maryland

MARCEL DEKKER, INC.   New York and Basel

Library of Congress Cataloging in Publication Data

Carter, Walter H., Jr. [Date]
    Regression analysis of survival data in cancer
chemotherapy.

    (Statistics, textbooks and monographs; v. 44)
    Includes index.
    1. Cancer--Chemotherapy--Evaluation--Statistical
methods. 2. Regression analysis. 3. Chemotherapy,
Combination--Evaluation--Statistical methods.
I. Wampler, Galen L., [Date]. II. Stablein,
Donald M., [Date]. III. Title. IV. Series.
[DNLM: 1. Neoplasms--Drug therapy. 2. Regression
analysis. QZ 267 C3255r]
RC271.C5C3274 1983   616.99'4061   82-17945

MARCEL DEKKER, INC.
270 Madison Avenue, New York, New York 10016

Current printing (last digit):
10 9 8 7 6 5 4 3 2 1

PRINTED IN THE UNITED STATES OF AMERICA

I would like to dedicate this book to

> Lyle Hansbrough, who died of leukemia before effective chemotherapy was available

> Carolyn Lacy, who was unsuccessfully treated with combination chemotherapy for breast cancer and died of her disease after suffering from the side effects of such treatment

> Duncan Gibb, who initially responded to combination chemotherapy for his lung cancer but ultimately relapsed and died of his disease

> Bob Priode, whose lymphoma is in remission as a result of combination chemotherapy

It is my hope that the techniques presented in this text will play a useful role in decreasing the number of those, like Lyle Hansbrough, Carolyn Lacy, and Duncan Gibb, for whom no effective therapy existed and increasing the number of those who, like Bob Priode, can benefit from the treatment of their disease.

Walter H. Carter, Jr.

Preface

Currently the clinical study of chemotherapeutic agents can be divided into three phases. The objects of phase I are the determination of the maximum level of drug(s) above which excessive toxicity occurs and the description of the types of toxicities seen. The primary goal of phase II is to determine if there is clinical activity in the subtoxic dosage range determined as a result of phase I studies. During this phase interest is still focused on toxicity, but only secondarily. Finally, phase III consists of a comparative study, the object of which is to determine if a new drug or combination which has shown promise as a result of phase II study offers improved results when compared to the standard treatment. Significant in this approach is the lack of any systematic effort to determine optimal levels of treatment. The approach used assumes that the optimum dose is the dose just under a toxic dose. This approach is more valid for a single drug than for combinations in which toxic doses exist for all of the many combinations of different dose ratios.

In clinical drug studies the treatment of interest should be the optimum. If a trial is performed to evaluate the efficacies of drug combinations, any comparison other than a comparison of the combinations employed at their optimal levels is

misleading. While the hypothesis of no treatment difference
can always be tested, if the optima are not used, such procedures add little, if any, information about the best way to
treat with given combinations. There are implicit logical
problems associated with the current methods of combination
evaluations. These result from not considering the response
surface described by the joint effects of the drugs in combination. It is often the case when treatments are being compared
that an entire combination is rejected, possibly never to be
considered again, as a result of the inferiority of the particular treatment levels used.

An example from the clinical literature involving the use
of antacids to treat peptic ulcer disease (to be discussed in
Chap. 1), points to the misleading nature of trials involving
doses other than the optimum and to the difficult problem of
locating the optimum. In this example, presence or absence of
response, rather than time to response, is the outcome variable.
There are other interesting and sometimes tragic illustrations
in the clinical literature of the failure to attend to the underlying response surfaces. Retrolental fibroplasia, which
accompanies oxygen therapy of premature infants, is a disorder
leading to blindness. James and Lanman* note that failure to
relate the percentages of both survival and ocular problems
simultaneously to the dosage of oxygen has caused years of con-
troversy as to the proper mode of treatment.

The problems the cancer chemotherapist faces are similar,
though not identical, to those in the examples. The existence
of multiple drugs in the combination substantially increases
the dimensions of the treatment space and the magnitude of the
problem. The presence of multiple sources of toxicity, multiple pathways of activity, and multiple mechanisms for beneficial

---

*James, S., and Lanman, J. (1976). History of oxygen therapy
and retrolental fibroplasia. *Pediatrics*, *57*, Supplement.

effects make the problem one that can be solved only through properly designed controlled clinical experiments.

Phase I and phase II studies are presently credited with assuring that near optimal treatment levels are used. These studies are in fact aimed at determining if a new regimen has potential efficacy at subtoxic doses rather than at finding the location of the optimum. Dosage selection for clinical trials is often dependent solely on clinical insight. Clinical insight, as the examples demonstrate, cannot always be trusted to determine the appropriate dosages for evaluation, even in the single-drug case. In effect, the problem of attaining optimum doses is not being dealt with rigorously. It will not disappear by essentially ignoring it; rather it will result in consistently suboptimal patient care.

The full thrust of this text is to indicate that the statistician, through the modeling approach, can effectively aid in the solution of these problems. Although the methods presented are illustrated primarily with examples from preclinical studies, it is felt that eventually they, or extensions of them, will find application in clinical studies. This will not be accomplished without difficulty. Modifications will have to be made. Toxic doses, for example, cannot be deliberately administered; this restriction limits the curvature of the visible response surface. Instead, constraint functions may have to be estimated as discussed in Chaps. 2 and 6 to allow only permissible levels of side effects.

Clinical trials, as performed today, are incapable of predicting regions of improved treatment. If the tested treatment levels are unsuccessful, modification of dosages for improvement of therapy is impossible on the basis of information gathered. Regression-based approaches for clinical experimentation can provide new information which should lead to improvements in the quality of care through the effective location of optimal treatment levels.

This book is being written at the stage when response-surface methodology as applied to the biomedical sciences is in its infancy. Many of the ideas and procedures suggested need further development. It seems important to collect at this time the information that has been accumulated up to now so that others can begin to utilize and perfect these experimental systems. To this end, we have included information that will allow readers to use these methods.

We gratefully acknowledge the help of the many individuals to whom we owe debts of gratitude. Eleanor D. Campbell aided in the development of the Appendix and is responsible for the analyses leading to many of the figures and tables included in the test. Vernon Williams assisted in the development of some of the computer programs used in the analysis of the data of the examples. Juanita Coon, Ersell Dortch, and Donnalee Coon carried out the experiments used to illustrate the analytical techniques. We would like to acknowledge the support of the Medical College of Virginia-Virginia Commonwealth University Cancer Center. Kim Saunders, Susan Woolford, and Jacqueline McGrath typed various drafts of the manuscript and we extend our gratitude to them. During the development of the analytical methods presented here we benefited from discussions with Professor Nathan Mantel and we are indebted to him. The Biometric Society, Cancer Research Editorial Office, American Society of Quality Control, and *Journal of Statistical Computation and Simulation* have given permission to include program listings and copies of figures and charts which appeared initially in their publications. The research which led to the development of the techniques presented in this text was partially supported by grant CA23333 from the National Cancer Institute.

Walter H. Carter, Jr.
Galen L. Wampler
Donald M. Stablein

Contents

1

The Rationale for Application of Regression Methods in Combination Cancer Chemotherapy

1.1 BACKGROUND INFORMATION

In the years since it was first demonstrated that drugs could be used effectively in the treatment of cancer, much research has been devoted to learning about their effective administration. The developments in this text are directly related to determinations of how to use drugs effectively in combination, rather than to the use of single-agent therapy. Although the examples and discussion involve combination therapy with cyto-toxic agents in the treatment of cancer, the methods discussed are applicable to any clinical or preclinical process where multiple independent variables, under the control of the investigator, affect the desired response.

In pursuing this topic one must first appreciate that locating the optimum for a combination differs considerably from optimizing a single agent. For a single-factor process one has substantial help from everyday experience to aid in the solution. With toxic chemotherapeutic agents the classical preclinical approach involves treating groups of animals at several different dosage levels. The optimum is then determined by visual inspection of the improvements in response of the treated groups relative to that of the control group.

In effect, this procedure corresponds to surveying a two-dimensional surface to determine the location of the maximum value
of the response variable. In Fig. 1.1 such a surface is dia-
gramed. The rising portion of the curve is attributable to the
beneficial effects of the drug; then the curve falls due to the
toxicity inherent in its use. The optimum is that point just
preceding where toxic effects exceed beneficial ones. As a
rule, the experiment described will be successful in finding
this optimum dose if the density of coverage of the experimental region is sufficient and the space contains the true optimum within its interior.

This process, though simple, is effective only when a
single drug is considered. Adding a second drug causes the
scope of the problem to increase immediately and leads to the
examination of Fig. 1.2. All possible combinations of the
drugs A and B can be depicted in the positive quadrant of such

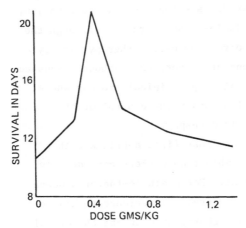

FIGURE 1.1. *Plot of dose-response curve for (±)-1,2-bis(3,5-
dioxopiperazin-1-yl)propane (ICRF-159) when given for treatment
of advanced solid L1210 leukemia in B6D2F$_1$ female mice. Treatment was started on day 7 after tumor inoculation and was given
as a single intraperitoneal treatment every fourth day until
death (maximum of three treatments).*

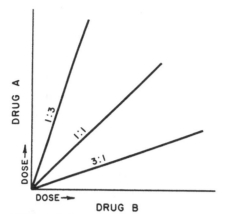

FIGURE 1.2.   Schematic diagram for ray design in two variables.

a graph. Assuming equal scaling, the rays designated 3:1, 1:1,
and 1:3 mark three different drug ratios among the set of all
possible ratios. Each drug ratio is essentially similar to a
single agent, as a two-dimensional curve like Fig. 1.1 describes
its dose-response effects. Optimizing any single ratio is therefore not a conceptually difficult problem. But as it is impossible to test all ratios, finding the correct ratio upon which
to perform the single-agent optimization is, from a practical
viewpoint, impossible. Further, it is easy to find a dosage
combination which causes toxicity just less than the acceptable
limit. The problem is that there is an entire set of such combinations, and it is unlikely that the beneficial effects associated with each are equivalent. Clearly, one requires different tools to survey a surface rather than a curve.

    The addition of a third drug, thereby adding another dimen-
sion, markedly increases the difficulty of optimum determination. Three two-drug planes exist in addition to all interior
points with three drugs present. Further, the surface to be
surveyed is now a four-dimensional one, and even if it is practical to run large enough experiments to adequately cover the
possible dose combinations, pictorial representation of the

results is no longer simple. Intuitive attempts at exploration
or extension of the one-dimensional solution become lost in the
dimensionality of the region.

Scientific exploration of four, five, or more drugs in combination becomes an exceptionally difficult problem. We know
of no published preclinical attempts to deal with problems this
large. Yet the routine administration of up to six drugs in
the clinical treatment of cancer is not uncommon.

Clearly, effective use of combinations, i.e., usage at
optimal levels, requires procedures directed toward determining those levels. In biologic systems use of suboptimum doses
even when only a single drug is administered is possible. An
example, although not with antineoplastic drugs, illustrates
the point. Hollander and Harlan [3], in a double-blind randomized study of the efficacy of antacid versus placebo in the
treatment of peptic ulcer, determined no benefit to antacid
treatment. Peterson et al. [6] performed a similar trial several years later and found a significant ($p < 0.005$) effect of
the antacid therapy. Although there were some differences between the trials (the latter used endoscopy to evaluate ulcer
healing), the most remarkable difference is that Peterson et
al. used the equivalent of a dose nearly eight times as large
as that used in the Hollander and Harlan trial. The first
study compared no treatment with inadequate treatment and concluded there was no difference. The second study greatly
increased the dosage. Thus an effective treatment was found,
but the question as to the optimal treatment level is still
open. Little information about the optimum dose is available
despite the effort, expense, and human costs for the described
controlled trials.

With drug combinations, additional factors must be considered. With two drugs, A and B, it is possible to administer
them simultaneously, with A preceding B, or with B preceding A.

With three drugs there are 13 such orderings; combinations of four drugs yield 81 orderings. The time interval between drug doses is an additional variable which could also be explicitly considered.

Confronted with the many possible ways to administer n drugs, a question that comes to mind is, "Do all these variations make a difference?" In considering this question, 24 of the possible permutations for sequential use of four drugs were tested. Table 1.1 shows the results of testing cyclophosphamide (C), vincristine (O), methotrexate (M), and 5-fluorouracil. (F). A single time interval of 24 hr was selected (T = 24 hr), as were single doses of each drug: C = 50 mg/kg, O = 0.5 mg/kg, M = 1.25 mg/kg, and F = 25 mg/kg; dosages of each well below the toxic range were considered in order to minimize toxic effects. The experiment was conducted in 20-g B6D2F$_1$ female mice, injecting each intraperitoneally (i.p.) with 10^5 L1210 cells 24 hr before the treatment began. There were eight mice per group. Results for triplicate experiments are shown. Using the median of the replicate experiments, increases in life span over controls from 6.6 to 12+ days occurred. It is well known that a one-log kill of these leukemic cells extends the life of the animal about two days. These results can, therefore, be extrapolated as leukemic cell kills of approximately 99.9% to over 99.9999%--almost a three-log difference. Clearly, if the object is to find factors which have a real effect on drug combination applications, one does not have to look far.

From the preceding, it is clear that many experiments over a long period of time would be required before all of the possible combinations of the presently known drugs and schedules of administration could be tested in the laboratory. This situation is further complicated by the continuous discovery of additional compounds with antitumor activity. Indeed, with the introduction of each new compound it can be argued that we

TABLE 1.1. *Variations in Survival Time (in Days) as a Function of Treatment Sequence*

Treatment	Exp. 1	Exp. 2	Exp. 3
Control	8.3 + 0.2	7.9 ± 0.1	7.4 ± 0.2
C(24)O(24)M(24)F[a]	15.5 ± 0.3	15.4 ± 0.7	16.8 ± 0.9
C(24)O(24)F(24)M	15.0 ± 0.5	15.9 ± 0.3	16.0 ± 0.5
C(24)M(24)O(24)F	14.2 ± 0.4	14.5 ± 1.3	15.6 ± 0.6
C(24)M(24)F(24)O	14.8 ± 0.4	15.2 ± 0.9	16.1 ± 0.7
C(24)F(24)O(24)M	14.6 ± 0.5	15.6 ± 0.5	16.4 ± 0.6
C(24)F(24)M(24)O	14.8 ± 0.5	15.8 ± 0.7	16.6 + 0.7
O(24)C(24)M(24)F	16.6 ± 1.2	17.0 ± 1.8	16.5 ± 0.5
O(24)C(24)F(24)M	---	16.2 ± 0.4	16.0 ± 0.4
O(24)M(24)C(24)F	16.4 ± 0.2	17.0 ± 0.9	18.3 + 1.5
O(24)M(24)F(24)C	18.3 ± 0.8	19.4 ± 0.8	18.9 ± 0.7
O(24)F(24)C(24)M	18.8 ± 0.9	20.3 + 1.8	20.0 ± 1.7
O(24)F(24)M(24)C	16.5 ± 0.7	17.8 ± 0.6	18.6 + 1.0
M(24)C(24)O(24)F	16.8 + 1.0	22.3 ± 3.4	17.9 ± 0.6
M(24)C(24)F(24)O	11.0 ± 0.5	17.4 ± 0.6	17.3 + 0.9
M(24)O(24)C(24)F	18.0 + 1.6	16.8 ± 0.8	16.8 ± 0.5
M(24)O(24)F(24)C	18.3 + 0.6	21.3 ± 2.5	17.5 ± 0.7
M(24)F(24)C(24)O	19.6 ± 1.1	19.3 ± 0.7	---
M(24)F(24)O(24)C	16.6 ± 0.9	18.5 ± 0.9	18.0 + 0.7
F(24)C(24)O(24)M	18.6 ± 1.3	22.7 ± 2.5	19.5 ± 0.9
F(24)C(24)M(24)O	17.3 + 1.3	18.2 ± 0.5	20.6 + 1.3
F(24)O(24)C(24)M	15.5 + 0.9	17.3 ± 0.6	17.9 ± 0.6
F(24)O(24)M(24)C	14.4 ± 0.5	16.8 ± 1.1	17.0 ± 0.4
F(24)M(24)C(24)O	16.8 ± 0.5	18.9 ± 1.5	21.7 ± 2.2
F(24)M(24)O(24)C	15.6 ± 0.4	21.4 ± 2.4	17.3 ± 0.7

[a]C = cyclophosphamide, 1 mg per mouse (50 mg/kg)
 O = vincristine, 10 μg per mouse (0.5 mg/kg)
 M = methotrexate, 25 μg per mouse (1.25 mg/kg)
 F = 5-fluorouracil, 0.5 mg per mouse (25 mg/kg)

Treatments were given sequentially on days 1 to 4 following tumor inoculation of 10^5 L1210 cells i.p. into B6D2F$_1$ female mice.

fall further behind in the research required to support the use
of combinations in clinical studies. Few papers have appeared
in the literature reporting on the use of three or more drugs
in combination. However, as already noted, it is not unusual
to see that four, five, or more drugs have been used in combination clinically. The clinical use of drugs in combination
prior to adequate animal studies is understandable, in light
of the complexity associated with testing combinations. However, there are likely to be unfortunate consequences of such
a strategy. Specifically, once a combination has been shown
to be ineffective its use is likely to be discontinued. However, there is the very real possibility that the failure of
the combination is due to the use of improper dosage levels,
not to the combination's being truly ineffective. Thus, there
is a need for an experimental procedure, incorporating the design and analysis of combination chemotherapy experiments,
which will yield information concerning optimality conditions.

Response-surface methodology (RSM) is a collection of
mathematical and statistical methods which has been developed
and used to aid in the solution of particular types of problems pertinent to scientific and engineering processes. The
methods include experimental design, statistical inference,
and mathematical optimization techniques, which when combined
enable the experimenter to make an efficient empirical exploration of the process on which interest is centered. This
approach to exploring relationships between variables has, to
date, found its greatest application in industrial settings.
In fact, its modern development was motivated by problems faced
in the chemical industry. Typically the problem faced in this
area is one of optimizing the yield of a particular process.
In such situations, for example, it is known that the yield of
the process is related to the levels of the input variables,
such as temperature, pressure, cooking time, etc., and it is

of interest to determine the level of each of these variables
associated with optimum yield.

The essence of a response surface approach is that a mathematical relationship (model) exists between the levels of
treatment and the outcome observed. Thus, one generally works
with causal models where the levels of treatment or design variables are controllable by the researcher. In RSM the treatment variables appear in a regression sense as opposed to an
analysis of variance sense. By this it is meant that the model
is parameterized in such a way that the actual levels of treatment are related to the survival experience so that the effects
of different levels of treatment can be predicted. This is as
opposed to a parameterization whereby only comparisons between
different treatment groups are permitted. The importance of
this distinction lies in the fact that once the levels of treatment are related to the treatment outcome in a regression sense,
RSM can be used to explore the resulting response surfaces and
obtain information not forthcoming from other analyses.

There are several stages to the usual response–surface
analysis:

1. Experimental design
2. Model selection and parameter estimation
3. Model verification
4. Exploration of the fitted response surface

These phases of a response surface analysis are given in the
chronological order performed once it has been determined to
employ the RSM experimental approach. From the point of view
of statistical development, it is more natural to consider the
estimation of the model parameters prior to the development of
the experimental design. This follows since once the estimation procedure has been established and estimators determined,
the statistical properties of the estimators as a function of
the location of the design points can be ascertained. As a

result, it is often possible to determine the placement of experimental points in such a manner as to optimize certain desirable properties of the estimators.

Unfortunately, the application of these techniques to problems faced by biomedical researchers has been limited. This conclusion is documented and discussed by Mead and Pike [5]. Specifically, in his discussion of Mantel's [4] paper, Box [2] early on suggested the potential usefulness of regression analysis in gaining an understanding of the relationship between levels of treatment and their effect. For example, with an appropriate model it would be possible to gain an indication of the effect of the drugs in different ratios and doses than those used in the experiment described by Mantel. Box further suggested that a more realistic analysis might include modeling the relationship among treatment levels and various manifestations of toxicity in addition to the endpoint of major interest, i.e., survival. Once these models had been developed and their predictive ability verified it would then be possible to determine treatment levels associated with maximum survival, subject to constraints placed on the incidence or levels of the various measures of toxicity.

Eight years after Box suggested the usefulness of regression methods in analyzing data from combination chemotherapy experiments, Addelman, Gaylor, and Bohrer [1] devised an experimental scheme for estimating the optimal combination of two drugs. Historically, theirs is the initial paper reporting on the use of such methods in this area of cancer research. The procedure is such that at most three experiments must be performed. The first experiment uses three doses from within the effective range of each of the individual drugs and nine combinations arrived at by considering three different ratios between the levels of the two drugs, in a manner not unlike that described earlier. The data described from this experiment are then analyzed by fitting the quadratic function

$$y = \beta_0 + \beta_1 x_1 + \beta_2 x_2 + \beta_{11} x_1^2 + \beta_{22} x_2^2 + \beta_{12} x_1 x_2$$

where

y = lifespan of the experimental subject

$x_i = \log\left(\dfrac{x_{iL}}{100} + \text{dose level of compound i, mg/kg}\right)$, $i = 1, 2$

x_{iL} = lower extreme of effective range of compound i

$\beta\text{'s}$ = unknown constants (to be estimated from the data) which parameterize the model

After some initial data selection, performed to improve the predictability of the regression function, the unknown model parameters are estimated by the method of least squares. After the parameter estimation has been accomplished, the underlying response surface is explored and an optional combination is estimated. Using the information obtained as a result of the analysis of the first experiment, a second experiment is performed. The authors give conditions under which portions of the original data can be combined with those obtained as a result of the second experiment and then used to reestimate the parameters of the quadratic dose-response model. Again, optimal levels of treatment are estimated from an exploration of the response surface. The criteria for determining if this second estimated optimum should be considered as the final estimate are then developed. If it is determined that a third experiment is necessary, procedures similar to those utilized after the second experiment can be used to determine how data from the prior experiments are to be used in fitting the quadratic relationship between dosage levels and survival time. Unless there is some indication that the optimal combination estimated after the third experiment is unrealistic, the search procedure is terminated. Unfortunately, the

authors illustrated their procedures with hypothetical data.
Thus they could report neither how well their model related
treatment levels to survival times nor the accuracy of the
estimates of optimal dosage. Further, the skewed nature of
many survival distributions may affect the accuracy of pre-
dictions based on a linear model.

1.2 CONCLUSION

In summary, the visual or intuitive approach to locating optimal treatment combinations fails when the dimensionality of
both the treatment and response spaces become large. The considerable variability that exists within experimental situations makes interpretation of the results difficult. Additionally, the required multidimensional interpolation makes successful estimation of the optima nearly impossible. Other techniques for dosage optimization and analysis are clearly required.

In the following chapters the application of RSM to the
problems of determining combined modality therapy of cancer
will be developed and illustrated. It should be noted that
these techniques are general and therefore apply to combinations of drugs and radiation therapy or investigation of time
intervals. Obviously they can be useful in determining levels
of treatment in any disease when treatment is a quantitative
variable. However, in this text attention will be restricted
to the treatment of cancer with combinations of drugs, without
the loss of generality.

REFERENCES

1. Addelman, S., Gaylor, D. W., and Bohrer, Q. E. (1966).
   Sequences of combination chemotherapy experiments.
   Biometrics, 22, 730-746.

2. Box, G. E. P. (1958). In Discussion of experimental design in combination chemotherapy. *Ann. N.Y. Acad. Sci.,
   76,* 909-931.

3. Hollander, D., and Harlan, J. (1973). Antacids vs. placebo in peptic ulcer therapy: A controlled double-blind investigation. *J. Amer. Med. Assoc.*, *226*, 1181–1185.

4. Mantel, N. (1958). Experimental design in combination chemotherapy. *Ann. N.Y. Acad. Sci.*, *76*, 909–931.

5. Mead, R., and Pike, D. J. (1975). A review of response surface methodology from a biometrics viewpoint. *Biometrics*, *31*, 803–852.

6. Peterson, W., Sturdevant, R., Frankl, H., Richardson, C., Isenberg, J., Elashoff, J., Sones, J., Gross, R., McCallum, R., and Fordtran, J. (1977). Healing of duodenal ulcer with an antacid regimen. *New Eng. J. Med.*, *297*, 341–345.

2

The Logistic Regression Model

2.1 INTRODUCTION

In this chapter the logistic regression model will be introduced, and how this model can be used to relate treatment
levels to their effects will be indicated. It will be seen
that this approach is general in that it can be used to study
the combination of any number of treatment modalities, whether
they be a number of different drugs, drugs and radiation therapy, drugs used at different schedules, etc. Following the
development of the model, its use in analyzing data from a
single-drug experiment and a two-drug combination experiment
will be illustrated. Finally, the use of this model in situations where more than one treatment effect is of interest will
be explored.

2.2 DEVELOPMENT OF THE LOGISTIC REGRESSION MODEL

It is well known that when effective cytotoxic agents are used,
either singly or in combination, in the treatment of disease,
the chances of a favorable treatment outcome, however defined,
improve with increasing levels of treatment until the optimal
level of treatment is exceeded. From that point on in the
treatment space the chances of a favorable outcome decline due

to the toxicity associated with the treatment. Such a relationship is described in Fig. 2.1. In this figure the abscissa
represents treatment which could include combinations of agents.
This representation allows the figure to be drawn in two dimensions. Otherwise it would require a (k + 1)-dimensional figure
to describe such a relationship when k treatment modalities are
combined. Thus, a function which takes on values between 0 and
1 and which is capable of assuming such a shape is required in
order to effectively model this kind of relationship. The
logistic function quadratic in its argument satisfies these
requirements. Under this model the relationship between the
dose x of a single drug and the probability p of a favorable
outcome is given by

$$p = \{1 + \exp[-(\beta_0 + \beta_1 x + \beta_{11} x^2)]\}^{-1}$$

where β_0, β_1, and β_{11} are unknown constants which parameterize
the model. Over an appropriate range of dosage levels the
model parameters can be interpreted as: β_0 is related to the
probability of a favorable outcome when x = 0; β_1 is related
to the therapeutic effect of the drug; and β_{11} is related to
the toxicity of the drug. (Without this last parameter the
logistic dose-response function would not be able to decrease

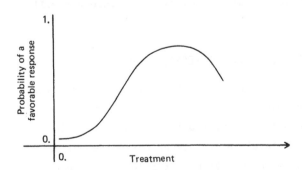

FIGURE 2.1. *Dose response curve for cytotoxic treatment.*

after the dose associated with the maximum probability of a favorable outcome was exceeded.)

This model is easily modified to handle treatments composed of a combination of therapeutic agents. When several agents are administered in combination there is the possibility of interactions between the various components of the treatment mixture. It is possible to account for such phenomena by including additional parameters in the model. For example, consider a three-drug combination. The model could then be written as

$$p = [1 + \exp(-\underline{x}'\underline{\beta})]^{-1}$$

where

$$\underline{x}'\underline{\beta} = \beta_0 + \beta_1 x_1 + \beta_2 x_2 + \beta_3 x_3 + \beta_{11} x_1^2 + \beta_{22} x_2^2 + \beta_{33} x_3^2$$
$$+ \beta_{12} x_1 x_2 + \beta_{13} x_1 x_3 + \beta_{23} x_2 x_3 + \beta_{123} x_1 x_2 x_3$$

and

x_1 = function of dose of drug 1

x_2 = function of dose of drug 2

x_3 = function of dose of drug 3

β_0 = unknown parameter associated with effect of treatment at 0 level of each drug

β_1 = unknown parameter associated with effect of drug 1

β_2 = unknown parameter associated with effect of drug 2

β_3 = unknown parameter associated with effect of drug 3

β_{11} = unknown parameter associated with toxicity of drug 1

β_{22} = unknown parameter associated with toxicity of drug 2

β_{33} = unknown parameter associated with toxicity of drug 3

β_{12} = unknown parameter associated with interaction between drugs 1 and 2

β_{13} = unknown parameter associated with interaction between drugs 1 and 3

β_{23} = unknown parameter associated with interaction
      between drugs 2 and 3

β_{123} = unknown parameter associated with the interaction
      among all three drugs

Once the form of the model has been decided, the method of
maximum likelihood can be used to estimate the model parameters.
The likelihood function is given by

$$L = C \prod_{i=1}^{G} P_i^{n_i}(1 - P_i)^{g_i - n_i}$$

where

C = constant independent of unknown parameters

G = number of treatment groups

P_i = probability of favorable outcome associated with ith
      treatment group

n_i = number of animals in ith group experiencing favorable
      outcome

g_i = number of animals in ith group

As a result of the assumption that the logistic model can be
used to describe the underlying dose response surface, it follows that

$$P_i = [1 + \exp(-\underline{x}_i'\underline{\beta})]^{-1}$$

where $\underline{x}_i'\underline{\beta}$ is determined as above. Upon differentiating $\ell n\ L$
with respect to the unknown parameters and equating the results
to 0, the following system of equations is obtained:

$$\sum_{i=1}^{G} g_i P_i - n_i = 0$$

$$\sum_{i=1}^{G} x_{ji}(g_i P_i - n_i) = 0$$

$$\sum_{i=1}^{G} x_{ji} x_{\ell i} (g_i p_i - n_i) = 0 \qquad j, \ell = 1, 2, \ldots, k$$

where k = number of elements in treatment combination.

Once this system of simultaneous nonlinear equations is solved for the parameter estimates, the estimated dose response surface can be explored. The determination of the significance of the model parameters can be accomplished either by likelihood ratio tests or through use of the asymptotic normality of the maximum-likelihood estimators. In this manner it is possible to learn of the statistical significance of the individual drug effects, the interactions between drugs within the combination, and the drugs' toxicities. Before using the model for predictive purposes, it is important to test for the adequacy of the model. This can be accomplished in a straightforward manner by comparing the observed number of favorable outcomes to that predicted by the model, i.e., compare n_i to $g_i \hat{p}_i$ for each of the treatment groups. ($\hat{p}_i$ is used to denote the estimate of p_i obtained by substituting the vector of parameter estimates $\underline{\hat{\beta}}$ for $\underline{\beta}$ in the expression for p_i.) The statistic

$$\chi^2 = \sum_{i=1}^{G} \frac{(n_i - g_i \hat{p}_i)^2}{g_i \hat{p}_i (1 - \hat{p}_i)}$$

is asymptotically distributed as a χ^2 random variable with $G - m$ degrees of freedom, where m is the number of parameters in the model; the statistic can be used to test for the adequacy of the model. If the model fit is inadequate, i.e., if there are discrepancies between the observed and predicted numbers of favorable treatment outcomes in the treatment groups, a large value of χ^2 can be expected. Thus, to test for statistically significant lack of fit one would compare χ^2 to $\chi^2_{1-\alpha, G-m}$, the $100(1 - \alpha)$ percentile of the χ^2 distribution with $G - m$ degrees of freedom. If χ^2 exceeds $\chi^2_{1-\alpha, G-m}$, there is an indication of

significant model inadequacy at the 100α% level of significance.
If $\chi^2 \leq \chi^2_{1-\alpha,G-m}$, there is no indication of model inadequacy
and further exploration of the underlying dose response surface
is reasonable. It is worth mentioning here that since any model
fitted to the data is likely to be artificial, it should not be
anticipated to fit too well. Indeed, the fact that a statistical test shows that a model fits the data is probably as indicative of the use of an inadequate sample size as it is indicative
of the choice of the proper model. As a result, all we expect
from a modeling approach is that it provide a reasonable guide
for learning about the treatment combination under consideration.

Notice that the estimated probability of a favorable outcome for treatment $\underline{x}$,

$$\hat{p} = [1 + \exp(-\underline{x}'\hat{\underline{\beta}})]^{-1}$$

is maximized when $\underline{x}'\hat{\underline{\beta}}$ is maximized. Thus, it follows that the
levels of treatment which maximize the estimated chance of a
favorable outcome can be obtained by maximizing $\underline{x}'\hat{\underline{\beta}}$ with respect to $\underline{x}$. If the experimental region contains toxic treat-
ments, an optimization of $\underline{x}'\hat{\underline{\beta}}$ with no restrictions on the treatment variables other than nonnegativeness will probably suffice;
a treatment so determined cannot have any very important toxicity, or it would not be an optimal treatment. However, if the
treatment space which defined the experiment is too narrow to
include toxic treatments, such a maximization could well lead
to levels of the treatment variables outside the region of experimentation and hence outside the region for which the representation of the response is accurate. In such a situation, it
would not be surprising to have significant toxicity associated
with the optimal treatment so determined. To avoid such an
occurrence, either the method of ridge analysis developed by
Hoerl [4] and refined by Draper [3] or the direct-optimization
method described by Nelder and Mead [5] could be used to

optimize $\underline{x}'\hat{\underline{\beta}}$, subject to the constraint that the solution must be in the region of the experiment and thus in the region for which the model gives an adequate explanation of the data.

2.3 CONFIDENCE REGION ABOUT THE OPTIMAL TREATMENT COMBINATION

Using a technique discussed by Box and Hunter [1] and the asymptotic properties of maximum-likelihood estimators it is possible to estimate a $100(1 - \alpha)\%$ confidence region for the optimal treatment combination. With the logistic model, the probability of a favorable outcome is related to treatment levels through the expression $\underline{x}'\underline{\beta}$ in such a manner that if it is a full quadratic

$$\frac{\partial \underline{x}'\underline{\beta}}{\partial x_i} = \beta_i + 2\beta_{ii}x_i + \sum_{\substack{j=1 \\ j \neq i}}^{k} \beta_{ij}x_j \qquad i = 1, 2, \ldots, k$$

where k = number of drugs in treatment combination. Under the assumption that the model is correct the true optimal dosage levels $(\xi_1, \xi_2, \ldots, \xi_k)$ must satisfy the expression

$$\beta_i + 2\beta_{ii}\xi_i + \sum_{\substack{j=1 \\ j \neq i}}^{k} \beta_{ij}\xi_j = 0 \qquad i = 1, 2, \ldots, k$$

Let δ_i be the maximum likelihood estimator of the left-hand side of the above equation, i.e.,

$$\delta_i = \hat{\beta}_i + 2\hat{\beta}_{ii}\xi_i + \sum_{\substack{j=1 \\ j \neq i}}^{k} \beta_{ij}\xi_j$$

Consider $\underline{\delta}$, the $k \times 1$ vector composed of the δ_i, $i = 1, 2, \ldots,$ k. Based on the asymptotic properties of the maximum-likelihood estimators it follows that

$$\underline{\delta} \overset{asy}{\cap} N(\underline{0}, V)$$

where the elements of V are the variances and covariances of the elements of $\underline{\delta}$. As a result of this asymptotic distribution it follows that

$$\underline{\delta}'V^{-1}\underline{\delta} \overset{asy}{\cap} \chi_k^2$$

Any values of $(\xi_1, \xi_2, \ldots, \xi_k)$ satisfying the inequality $\underline{\delta}'V^{-1}\underline{\delta} \leq \chi_{k,1-\alpha}^2$, where $\chi_{k,1-\alpha}^2$ is the $100(1 - \alpha)\%$ point of the χ^2 distribution with k degrees of freedom, fall into the $100(1 - \alpha)\%$ confidence region. It is informative to consider the special cases of a single drug and then a two-drug combination.

k = 1

In this case, under the assumption that the quadratic model is correct, the optimal treatment level ξ would be such that

$$\beta_1 + 2\beta_{11}\xi = 0$$

Here,

$$\delta_1 = \hat{\beta}_1 + 2\hat{\beta}_{11}\xi$$

and

$$
\begin{aligned}
V &= \text{var } \delta_1 \\
&= \text{var } \hat{\beta}_1 + 4\xi^2 \text{ var } \hat{\beta}_{11} + 4\xi \text{ cov}(\hat{\beta}_1, \hat{\beta}_{11})
\end{aligned}
$$

Let

$$\text{var } \hat{\beta}_1 = v_{11}$$
$$\text{var } \hat{\beta}_{11} = v_{22}$$
$$\text{cov}(\hat{\beta}_1, \hat{\beta}_{11}) = v_{12}$$

which can be obtained from the elements of the variance-covariance matrix of $\underline{\hat{\beta}}$. Then, if $\chi^2_{1-\alpha} = C$ the $100(1 - \alpha)\%$ confidence region about ξ is given by the solutions to

$$\underline{\delta} V^{-1} \underline{\delta} = \frac{(\hat{\beta}_1 + 2\hat{\beta}_{11}\xi)^2}{v_{11} + 4\xi^2 v_{22} + 4\xi v_{12}} \leq C$$

or

$$(4\hat{\beta}_{11}^2 - 4Cv_{22})\xi^2 + (4\hat{\beta}_1\hat{\beta}_{11} - 4Cv_{12})\xi + (\hat{\beta}_1^2 - Cv_{11}) \leq 0$$

$k = 2$

Given that the true model is quadratic, the optimal treatment levels (ξ_1, ξ_2) satisfy

$$\beta_1 + 2\beta_{11}\xi_1 + \beta_{12}\xi_2 = 0$$
$$\beta_2 + 2\beta_{22}\xi_2 + \beta_{12}\xi_1 = 0$$

Thus,

$$\delta_1 = \hat{\beta}_1 + 2\hat{\beta}_{11}\xi_1 + \hat{\beta}_{12}\xi_2$$
$$\delta_2 = \hat{\beta}_2 + 2\hat{\beta}_{22}\xi_2 + \hat{\beta}_{12}\xi_1$$

and

$$\text{var } \underline{\delta} = V$$
$$= \begin{bmatrix} \text{var } \delta_1 & \text{cov}(\delta_1, \delta_2) \\ \text{cov}(\delta_1, \delta_2) & \text{var } \delta_2 \end{bmatrix}$$

has as its elements

$$\text{var } \delta_1 = v_{11} + 4\xi_1^2 v_{33} + \xi_2^2 v_{55} + 4\xi_1 v_{13} + 2\xi_2 v_{15}$$
$$+ 4\xi_1 \xi_2 v_{35}$$
$$\text{var } \delta_2 = v_{22} + 4\xi_2^2 v_{44} + \xi_1^2 v_{55} + 4\xi_2 v_{24} + 2\xi_1 v_{25}$$
$$+ 4\xi_1 \xi_2 v_{45}$$

$$\text{cov}(\delta_1, \delta_2) = v_{12} + 2\xi_2 v_{14} + \xi_1 v_{15} + 2\xi_1 v_{23} + 4\xi_1 \xi_2 v_{34}$$
$$+ 2\xi_1^2 v_{35} + \xi_2 v_{25} + \xi_2^2 v_{45} + \xi_1 \xi_2 v_{55}$$

where

$$\text{var }\hat{\underline{\beta}} = \begin{bmatrix} v_{11} & v_{12} & v_{13} & v_{14} & v_{15} \\ v_{12} & v_{22} & v_{23} & v_{24} & v_{25} \\ v_{13} & v_{23} & v_{33} & v_{34} & v_{35} \\ v_{14} & v_{24} & v_{34} & v_{44} & v_{45} \\ v_{15} & v_{25} & v_{35} & v_{45} & v_{55} \end{bmatrix}$$

As a result, the $100(1 - \alpha)\%$ confidence region about (ξ_1, ξ_2) is defined to be all values of (ξ_1, ξ_2) which satisfy

$$\underline{\delta}' v^{-1} \underline{\delta} \leq \chi^2_{2,1-\alpha}$$

2.4 EXAMPLES

To illustrate the methods discussed, two examples will be given. The first involves the analysis of data resulting from the use of cyclophosphamide (CTX) in the treatment of murine P388 leukemia. In this experiment each of 64 BDF_1 female mice was injected intraperitoneally with 10^6 P388 cells. Mice were randomly divided into an untreated control group (16 animals) and six treatment groups (8 animals per group). Treatment began seven days after the P388 injection. The time of death of each animal was recorded. Table 2.1 contains, among other information, the treatment levels and survival times associated with each animal.

To account for the observed drug toxicity, the following model was used:

Probability of at least 21-day survival
$$= \{1 + \exp[-(\beta_0 + \beta_1 x + \beta_{11} x^2)]\}^{-1}$$

where

TABLE 2.1. *Survival Data and Goodness of Fit Statistics for the Cyclophosphamide Experiment*

Treatment (mg/kg)		Animals living at least 21 days		
CTX	Survival times (days)	Observed frequency	Predicted frequency	Group χ^2
0.0	$9(9)^a,10(6),11(1)$	0	0.0081	0.0081
65.7	$9,10,13,18,20,23,25(2)$	3	2.3286	0.2730
92.0	$9(2),12,23(2),25,26,82^+$	5	5.8615	0.4737
164.0	$27,28,29,30(2),36(2),42$	8	7.8437	0.1594
230.0	$30(2),34,35,36,38,40,32^+$	8	7.7943	0.2111
296.0	$9,13(2),29,36,41(2),100^+$	5	5.0460	0.0011
414.0	$8(2),9(2),10,12,13,17$	0	0.0001	0.0001

[a]The number in parentheses indicates the number of deaths on that day.
[+]Censored observation.

$$x = \text{dose (mg/kg) of CTX}$$

β_0, β_1, β_{11} = unknown constants which parameterize the model

The estimates of the model parameters obtained by maximizing the previously defined likelihood function, their standard deviations, and p values associated with the tests of their significance appear in Table 2.2. From the table it can be concluded that each of the parameters is significantly different from zero. By considering the functional form of the model, it follows that treatment factors with positive coefficients act to increase the probability of surviving at least 21 days. Thus, it can be concluded that for the dosage range considered, CTX has a significant effect in increasing the probability of at least 21-day survival, but it is also a drug with significant toxicity.

In order to use the predictive ability of the model to estimate the dosage level which maximizes the estimated probability of at least 21-day survival, it is first necessary to gain an indication of the adequacy of the model as a predictor. As discussed in Sect. 2.2, the χ^2 statistic is useful in making such a determination. The observed and predicted numbers of

TABLE 2.2. *Parameter Estimates, Tests of Significance, and Covariance Matrix for the Single Drug (CTX) Experiment*

Parameter	Maximum-likelihood estimate	Significance
β_0	7.5880	0.0049
β_1	−0.1232	0.0036
β_{11}	0.3235×10^{-3}	0.0044

$$\text{var } \hat{\underline{\beta}} = \begin{bmatrix} 0.8595 \times 10^{1} & -0.1313 & 0.3488 \times 10^{-3} \\ -0.1313 & 0.2090 \times 10^{-2} & -0.5627 \times 10^{-5} \\ 0.3488 \times 10^{-3} & -0.5627 \times 10^{-5} & 0.1528 \times 10^{-7} \end{bmatrix}$$

animals surviving 21 days or longer in each treatment group are given in Table 2.1, along with each treatment group's contribution to the total χ^2. From these, the value of χ^2 with 4 degrees of freedom is calculated to be 1.13, with an associated p value of 0.89. Accordingly, there is no evidence of statistically important lack of fit. As a result it is reasonable to use the model to estimate the optimal treatment combination.

In the previous section it was indicated that the optimum dose could be estimated by maximizing $\underline{x}'\hat{\underline{\beta}}$ with respect to $\underline{x}$. For this example, therefore, we require the value of x which maximizes $-0.0003235x^2 + 0.1232x - 7.588$. It follows that the estimated optimal level is x = 190.4 mg/kg of CTX. At this level, we would predict from the model that 98.4% of all treated animals could survive at least 21 days. This is in relatively close agreement with the experimental data. Using the technique discussed in Sect. 2.3 and the information in Table 2.2, the estimated 95% confidence interval about the optimal dosage ξ of CTX is given by 143.9 mg/kg $\leq \xi \leq$ 252.8 mg/kg. The estimated relationship between the probability of surviving at least 21 days and the dosage level of CTX is plotted in Fig. 2.2.

The second example involves the analysis of data resulting from the use of CTX and doxorubicin (ADR) in murine P388 leukemia. In this experiment each of 128 BDF_1 female mice was injected intraperitoneally with 10^6 P388 cells. Mice were randomly divided into 16 treatment groups (eight mice per group), including an untreated control group. Treatment began seven days after the P388 injection. The time of death of each animal was recorded and the experiment was terminated after 100 days. Table 2.3 contains, among other information, the treatment level and survival time associated with each animal.

Because of the potentially toxic nature of each drug and an interest in determining whether or not the drugs interacted, the following model was used:

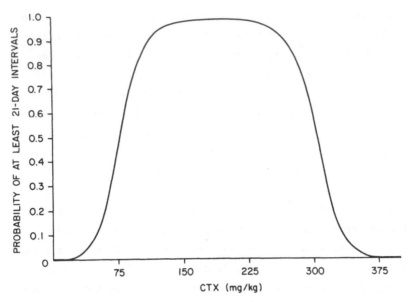

FIGURE 2.2. Estimated dose response curve for CTX treatment of advanced P388 leukemia.

Probability of at least 20-day survival =

$$\{1 + \exp[-(\beta_0 + \beta_1 x_1 + \beta_2 x_2 + \beta_{11} x_1^2 + \beta_{22} x_2^2 + \beta_{12} x_1 x_2)]\}^{-1}$$

where

x_1 = dose (mg/kg) of CTX
x_2 = dose (mg/kg) of ADR

The maximum-likelihood estimates of the model parameters, their variance-covariance matrix, and p values associated with the test of their significance based on their asymptotic normality appear in Table 2.4. As in the previous example, it is important to verify the adequacy of the model as a predictor prior to exploring the response surface it describes. When the χ^2 test of fit is performed it yields a test statistic of 20.6 with 10 degrees of freedom. The p value associated with this statistic is 0.024, which indicates a significant lack of fit.

TABLE 2.3. *Survival Data and Goodness of Fit Statistics for the CTX/ADR Experiment*

| Treatment (mg/kg) | | | Animals living at least 20 days | | |
CTX	ADR	Survival time (days)	Observed frequency	Predicted frequency	Group χ^2
0	0.0	9(2)[a],10(4),11(2)	0	0.1066	0.1080
149	0.0	10,12(2),18,26,29,36,62	4	4.3344	0.0563
223	0.0	19,20,24,25,26(3),33	7	5.9103	0.7691
335	0.0	13,14,16,20,24,38,39,47	5	5.2675	0.0398
0	2.8	9,10,11(5),12	0	0.3382	0.3532
0	4.2	10,11(4),12(2),19	0	0.4883	0.5200
0	6.3	10,11(3),12,15,16,66	1	0.6595	0.1916
149	2.8	30,32,34(2),40,62,64(2)	8	5.8933	2.8599
149	4.2	100+(3),12,32,33,36,42	7	6.2235	0.4363
149	6.3	100+(2),5,35,36,37,40,42	7	6.3326	0.3375
223	2.8	100+(2),15(2),16,17,33,43	4	6.8054	7.7450
223	4.2	100+(5),19,23,27	7	6.9451	0.0033
223	6.3	100+(3),15(2),16,33,40	5	6.9080	3.8607
335	2.8	100+(2),12,14,16,24,36,41	5	6.0217	0.7011
335	4.2	100+(5),31,36,46	8	6.0557	2.5686
335	6.3	100+(5),10,17,82	6	5.7099	0.0515

[a]The number in parentheses indicates the number of deaths on that day.

+Censored observations.

TABLE 2.4. *Parameter Estimates, Tests of Significance, and Covariance Matrix for the CTX/ADR Combination*

Parameter	Maximum-likelihood estimate	Significance
β_0	-4.3051	$p = 0.0023$
β_1	0.0422	$p = 0.0001$
β_2	0.5210	$p = 0.2051$
β_{11}	-0.8176×10^{-4}	$p = 0.0001$
β_{22}	-349.5×10^{-4}	$p = 0.4871$
β_{12}	-7.7618×10^{-4}	$p = 0.4627$

$$\text{var } \hat{\underline{\beta}} = \begin{bmatrix} 1.9885 & 0.1277 \times 10^{-1} & -0.3756 & 0.1876 \times 10^{-4} & 0.1296 \times 10^{-1} & 0.1117 \times 10^{-2} \\ 0.1277 \times 10^{-1} & 0.1068 \times 10^{-3} & 0.1737 \times 10^{-2} & -1.9617 \times 10^{-7} & -0.2395 \times 10^{-4} & -0.6393 \times 10^{-5} \\ -0.3756 & 0.1737 \times 10^{-2} & 0.1691 & -0.1799 \times 10^{-5} & -0.1607 \times 10^{-1} & -0.2721 \times 10^{-3} \\ 0.1876 \times 10^{-4} & -1.9617 \times 10^{-7} & -0.1799 \times 10^{-5} & 4.3978 \times 10^{-10} & 2.6283 \times 10^{-8} & 5.8004 \times 10^{-9} \\ 0.1296 \times 10^{-1} & -0.2395 \times 10^{-4} & -0.1607 \times 10^{-1} & 2.6282 \times 10^{-8} & 0.2529 \times 10^{-2} & 0.3168 \times 10^{-5} \\ 0.1117 \times 10^{-2} & -0.6393 \times 10^{-5} & -0.2721 \times 10^{-3} & 5.8004 \times 10^{-9} & 0.3168 \times 10^{-5} & 0.1117 \times 10^{-5} \end{bmatrix}$$

Table 2.3 contains information which is useful in interpreting this result. The column labeled "Group χ^2" gives the contribution of each treatment group to the total χ^2. From this table it can be seen that with the exception of treatment group 11, there is good agreement between the observed and predicted number of at least 20-day survivors. Indeed, if treatment group 11 were deleted the subsequent value of χ^2 would become 12.9 with 9 degrees of freedom and have associated with it a p value of 0.17. However, the validity of such a posteriori reasoning is at best questionable. Important to the interpretation of the goodness of fit test as described in Sect. 2.2 is an appreciation of the fact that the distribution of the test statistic is approximately that of a χ^2 random variable with the quality of the approximation improving with increasing numbers of animals per treatment group. In the present example specifically, and in animal experiments in general, the number of animals per group is small enough to permit legitimate questioning of the appropriateness of using the percentage points of a χ^2 distribution in interpreting the test of fit. In a case such as this, the information in Table 2.3 which permits the comparison of the observed and predicted frequencies increases in importance. An additional, though related, indication of the strength of the estimated relationship between treatment levels and the probability of at least 20-day survival can be obtained from testing the hypothesis that the vector of model parameters equals 0, i.e., H_0: $\underline{\beta} = \underline{0}$. If this hypothesis were accepted, there would be no indication that there was a relationship between treatment levels and the probability of at least 20-day survival. For this example the likelihood-ratio test yields a p value less than 0.0001. Thus, the relationship between treatment and response is statistically significant. This result, combined with the information in Table 2.3, would appear to indicate that further exploration of the fitted response surface is justified.

Using the direct method of Nelder and Mead [5], the estimated optimal treatment is found to consist of a dose of 234 mg/kg of CTX and a dose of 4.8 mg/kg of ADR. At this level of treatment it is estimated that 87.2% of similarly diseased animals will live at least 20 days. Estimates of the effects of treatment at different dosage levels can be obtained from a plot of the underlying dose response surface. Since a two-drug combination is being considered, the dose response surface is three dimensional. One dimension is required to represent the response (the probability of surviving at least 20 days), while the other two dimensions are required to represent all possible dosage levels of the two drugs used in the treatment. The dimensionality of the surface makes it difficult to represent it graphically. However, by considering contours of constant response the dimensions can be decreased by one. Thus, for a two-drug combination the dose response surface can be represented in two dimensions. Figure 2.3 is such a plot, with increasing levels of the probability of surviving at least 20 days represented by increasingly darker shadings.

The asymptotic 95% confidence region about the optimal combination is given in Fig. 2.4. Unfortunately, the region is unbounded. For a detailed explanation of the conditions leading to such confidence regions the reader is referred to the paper by Box and Hunter [1]. These regions are highly dependent upon the experimental design used and the variability in the data. Box and Hunter give an example in which a 3^2 design was used to generate data for fitting a second-degree model. The confidence region about the optimum is of a similar shape to that given in Fig. 2.4. Merely by including six additional experimental points and reanalyzing the data, the resulting confidence interval was closed. The possibility of such an outcome, combined with the information already obtained in testing for the adequacy of the fit of the model, suggests that a

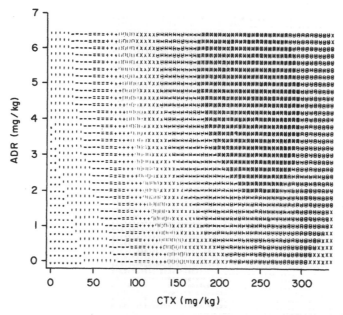

FIGURE 2.3. *Contours of constant probability of surviving at least 20 days, estimated for CTX/ADR treatment of advanced P388 leukemia. The range of estimated probability associated with each symbol is as follows:*

······	0.000 to 0.056	++++++	0.389 to 0.500
''''''	0.056 to 0.167	000000	0.500 to 0.611
------	0.167 to 0.278	XXXXXX	0.611 to 0.722
======	0.278 to 0.389	θθθθθθ	0.722 to 0.833
		&&&&&&	0.833 to 0.944
		⊕⊕⊕⊕⊕⊕	0.944 to 1.000

new experiment combining CTX and ADR over a wider range of dosage levels might yield improved results. At the very least, it would appear that our understanding of the two drugs in combination would be improved by augmenting the original experiment.

Further examples of confidence regions about the optimal dosage levels of drugs in combination are given in the following chapter.

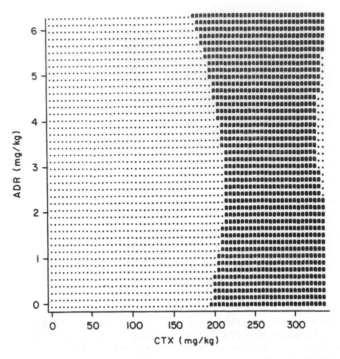

*FIGURE 2.4. Confidence region (95%) about optimal treatment
levels for CTX/ADR treatment of advanced P388 leukemia. Dosage
levels within the confidence region are indicated by the dark
symbol.*

2.5 CONSTRAINTS ON TREATMENT

In the previous section it was indicated that the experimental
region should be broad enough to contain toxic treatment combinations in order that the fitted dose response surface might
actually reflect the undesirable consequences of using treatment levels that are too high. While the reasons for this are
obvious, there are situations in which such experiments are not
feasible. Certainly, in a clinical situation involving combination therapy, treatment levels associated with lethal toxicity
would never be intentionally considered. Nevertheless, an
understanding of the underlying dose response surface is

essential to proper treatment. By modeling the incidence of undesirable outcomes, it is possible to estimate the levels of treatment associated with enabling the greatest predicted proportion of treated individuals to experience a favorable outcome while holding the incidence of undesirable side effects at or below a fixed level. Methods for accomplishing this will be discussed in this section.

Perhaps the most general way of accomplishing such an analysis is through the use of the multinomial logistic function to model the relationships between the various outcome categories and the levels of treatment. For simplicity, consider the situation in which it is possible to have the following four possible outcomes:

0_1: a favorable treatment response and an acceptable toxicity response
0_2: a favorable treatment response and an unacceptable toxicity response
0_3: an unfavorable treatment response and an acceptable toxicity response
0_4: an unfavorable treatment response and an unacceptable toxicity response

where, for example, a favorable treatment response in an animal study may be defined as surviving at least twice the median survival time of the untreated control group and an acceptable toxicity response may be defined as experiencing no more than a 10% weight loss as measured 14 days after treatment was administered. Under these circumstances, the likelihood function can be written as

$$L = C \prod_{i=1}^{G} p_{1i}^{n_{1i}} p_{2i}^{n_{2i}} p_{3i}^{n_{3i}} p_{4i}^{n_{4i}}$$

where

C = a constant independent of the model parameters

G = number of different treatment groups

p_{ji} = probability of an O_j, j = 1, 2, 3, 4 outcome in ith
treatment group (note that $p_{4i} = 1 - p_{1i} - p_{2i} - p_{3i}$)

g_i = number of subjects in ith treatment group

n_{ji} = number of O_j, j = 1, 2, 3, 4 outcomes in ith treatment group (note that $n_{4i} = g_i - n_{1i} - n_{2i} - n_{3i}$)

As a result of the assumption of an underlying multinomial logistic function,

$$p_{1i} = \frac{\exp(-\underline{x}'\underline{\beta}_1)}{1 + \Sigma_{i=1}^{3} \exp(-\underline{x}'\underline{\beta}_i)} \qquad p_{3i} = \frac{\exp(-\underline{x}'\underline{\beta}_3)}{1 + \Sigma_{i=1}^{3} \exp(-\underline{x}'\underline{\beta}_i)}$$

$$p_{2i} = \frac{\exp(-\underline{x}'\underline{\beta}_2)}{1 + \Sigma_{i=1}^{3} \exp(-\underline{x}'\underline{\beta}_i)} \qquad p_{4i} = \frac{1}{1 + \Sigma_{i=1}^{3} \exp(-\underline{x}'\underline{\beta}_i)}$$

The logic used in the determination of the form of $\underline{x}'\underline{\beta}_i$ parallels that given in Sect. 2.2. The parameter estimates are obtained by simultaneously solving the system of equations which result when the partial derivatives of L or ℓn L are equated to 0.

Once the parameters have been estimated, the goodness of fit of the model can be determined by comparing the expected number of responses in the outcome categories to the corresponding number of observed responses in each treatment group. The test statistic for the hypothesis of adequate fit is

$$\chi^2 = \sum_{i=1}^{G} \sum_{j=1}^{4} \frac{(n_{ji} - g_i \hat{p}_{ji})^2}{g_i \hat{p}_{ji}}$$

The distribution of this statistic approximates that of a χ^2 random variable with $3G - \gamma$ degrees of freedom, where γ equals the total number of parameters in the model. Thus, if $\chi^2 > \chi^2_{1-\alpha, 3G-\gamma}$ the hypothesis of adequate fit would be rejected at the $100\alpha\%$ level of significance. For the general case where there are m outcome categories the test statistic is given by

$$\chi^2 = \sum_{i=1}^{G} \sum_{j=1}^{m} \frac{(n_{ji} - g_i \hat{p}_{ji})^2}{g_i \hat{p}_{ji}}$$

which is asymptotically distributed as a χ^2 random variable
with $G(m - 1) - \gamma$ degrees of freedom.

Given that there is no indication of an inadequate fit,
the estimated response surface can be explored. The significance of individual parameters can be tested through use of the
likelihood-ratio criterion or by taking advantage of the asymptotic normality of the maximum-likelihood estimates. Further,
the treatment levels associated with the maximum estimated
probability of response in any one of the four outcome categories can be determined through use of the method of Nelder
and Mead [5].

As the number of model parameters increases, there must be
a concomitant increase in the number of treatment groups in the
experiment. A conservative rule of thumb to follow in these
situations requires the number of different treatment groups
to equal twice the number of parameters to be estimated. Thus,
for example, an experiment in two drugs to permit the estimation of the 18 parameters in a complete second-order logistic
function with four outcome categories would require 36 treatment groups. With 6 to 8 animals per treatment group the experiment would require 216 to 288 animals. A three-drug experiment to estimate the 30 parameters associated with the second-
order logistic function with only four outcome categories would
require 60 treatment groups and 360 to 480 animals. In the
general k-drug study, using a complete quadratic model with r
responses which can be categorized as acceptable or unacceptable, the number of treatment groups required can be written as
$2(2^r - 1)\left[\binom{k}{2} + 2k + 1\right]$. Thus, if either r or k is large this
approach quickly leads to experiments too large to be consid-
ered feasible.

One way of avoiding the problems associated with the increased parameterization which results from modeling polychotomous responses would be to determine which of the outcome groups is the most desirable. Using that set of treatment outcomes to define a favorable response, it would then be possible to use the methods of Sect. 2.2 to estimate and explore the underlying dose response surface. For example, consider the situation where the following outcome groups are under study:

O_1: acceptable survival, acceptable weight loss, acceptable white blood count

O_2: acceptable survival, acceptable weight loss, unacceptable white blood count

O_3: acceptable survival, unacceptable weight loss, acceptable white blood count

O_4: acceptable survival, unacceptable weight loss, unacceptable white blood count

O_5: unacceptable survival, acceptable weight loss, acceptable white blood count

O_6: unacceptable survival, acceptable weight loss, unacceptable white blood count

O_7: unacceptable survival, unacceptable weight loss, acceptable white blood count

O_8: unacceptable survival, unacceptable weight loss, unacceptable white blood count

Using O_1 to define a favorable response to treatment and O_2-O_8 to define a failure, it would be possible to relate, using the methods of Sect. 2.2, the levels of treatment to the probability of experiencing such an outcome.

If the treatment endpoints being recorded can be assumed independent of one another, fitting separate logistic regressions (Sect. 2.2) will result in a reduction of the number of parameters required to specify the model. For example, consider a two-drug combination where survival and hair loss are the endpoints of interest. Suppose further that a full second-degree model is required to describe the relationship between treatment levels and each of these endpoints. In this situation the multinomial approach would require 18 parameters, whereas modeling the two responses under the assumption of independence would require only 12 parameters. In general, fitting a full quadratic model in k drugs with r endpoints requires $[1 + 2k + \binom{k}{2}](2^r - 1)$ parameters. When the assumption of independence among the endpoints is reasonable, $[1 + 2k + \binom{k}{2}]r$ parameters are needed. Thus, from an experimental design point of view, much smaller experiments will suffice when the endpoints can be assumed to be independent of one another.

Wampler, Carter, and Williams [6] demonstrated this technique in a three-drug study with survival and day-12 weight loss as endpoints. These authors assumed independence of the endpoints and were able to show interesting relationships among the drug levels and survival when different levels of toxicity (day-12 weight loss) were tolerated.

2.6 LIMITATIONS OF THE USEFULNESS OF LOGISTIC MODELS

In this chapter logistic regression methods for relating treatment effects to treatment levels have been considered. A strength of these methods is that they can be used with categorical data, e.g., the treatment either led to an improvement in the subject's condition or it did not. However, if the response is a continuous variable, for example, survival time, its categorization could result in an important loss of information. For that reason, and since death is such a frequently used endpoint in cancer chemotherapy experiments, a regression-based approach to survival analysis is needed. The incorporation of time to response, particularly in the presence of some experimental survivors at the time of analysis will be discussed in the following chapter.

REFERENCES

1. Box, G. E. P., and Hunter, J. S. (1954). A confidence re-
    gion for the solution of a set of simultaneous equations
    with an application to experimental design. *Biometrika*,
    41, 190-199.

2. Cox, D. R. (1972). Regression models and life tables.
    J. Roy. Stat. Soc. B, *34*, 187-220.

3. Draper, N. R. (1963). Ridge analysis of response surfaces.
    Technometrics, *5*, 469-479.

4. Hoerl, A. E. (1959). Optimum solution of many variable
    equations. *Chem. Eng. Progr.*, *55*, 69-82.

5. Nelder, J. A., and Mead, R. A. (1965). A simplex method
    for function minimization. *Comp. J.*, *7*, 308-313.

6. Wampler, G. L., Carter, W. H., Jr., and Williams, V. R.
    (1978). Combination chemotherapy: Arriving at optimal
    treatment levels by incorporating side effect constraints.
    Cancer Treat. Rep., *62*, 333-340.

3

Proportional Hazards Analysis

3.1 INTRODUCTION

The logistic model discussed in the previous chapter is particularly applicable when the dependent variable for the experimental subject contains information only on whether or not a response occurred. One example might be the occurrence of a toxic event, such as significant alopecia, in treated individuals. In the example from the previous chapter, a success was defined as having a survival time twice the average of the control group. Thus, although the data could be analyzed after appropriate dichotomization of outcome, an important dimension of the response variable, namely time to death, has not been fully considered. It is the purpose of this chapter to explore the analysis of time to response or survival data when certain assumptions about the relationship of the treatment groups are applicable. It is important, first, to examine some of the basic concepts of survival theory.

Survival experience can be described by any of three functions: the death density function, the survival distribution, or the hazard function. The first function, the death density $f(t)$, defines the pattern of occurrence of failures by describing the instantaneous risk of death. Formally,

$$f(t) = \lim_{\Delta t \to 0^+} \frac{\Pr(t \leq T < t + \Delta t)}{\Delta t} \qquad (3.1)$$

The survivorship function, or survival distribution S(t), de-notes the probability of surviving at least as long as t. That is

$$S(t) = \Pr(T \geq t) \qquad (3.2)$$

and is a strictly nonincreasing function equaling 1 at T = 0.

The third function, which is very important in the devel-opment to follow, is the hazard function $\lambda(t)$. This function is defined as

$$\lambda(t) = \lim_{\Delta t \to 0^+} \frac{\Pr(t \leq T < t + \Delta t \mid T \geq t)}{\Delta t} \qquad (3.3)$$

The limiting probability of death in the interval (t, t + Δt), given survival to time t, is $\lambda(t) \Delta t$. Thus, the hazard func-tion denotes the instantaneous risk of death, providing death has not already occurred.

The above functions are substantially interrelated, the relationships being

$$f(t) = \frac{-dS(t)}{dt} \qquad (3.4)$$

$$S(t) = \exp\left(-\int_0^t \lambda(\mu) \, du\right) \qquad (3.5)$$

$$\lambda(t) = \frac{f(t)}{S(t)} \qquad (3.6)$$

Thus, specification of any one function implies the other two.

The development which follows depends on the hazard func-tion; therefore familiarity with this function is desirable. As has already been stated, the hazard function is a descrip-tion of the immediate risk of failure at every point in time. From another viewpoint, using Eq. (3.5) one can observe that the hazard function is the derivative of the natural logarithm of the survival distribution. Thus, the slope of the survival curve plotted on the natural log scale is the hazard function. If one considers the exponential distribution $S(t) = \exp(-\theta t)$, it is clear that the hazard function is constant, i.e., $\lambda(t) = \theta$. The exponential survival function supplies a simple model for a failure process, as there is no time-varying component in the process, i.e., the hazard function is independent of time. Other, more complicated, forms of the hazard function lead to well-known survival distributions. For example, if $\lambda(t) = \theta_0 \theta_1 t^{\theta_1 - 1}$, θ_0, $\theta_1 > 0$, the Weibull distribution with $S(t) = \exp(-\theta_0 t^{\theta_1})$ results. The hazard for the Weibull can be seen to either increase in time if $\theta_1 > 1$ or decrease in time if $\theta_1 < 1$.

Clearly, more complicated time-varying hazard forms are possible. For example, one can describe the risk of death in human populations. The hazard starts off high at birth and falls rapidly over the first year of life. In adolescence and early adulthood it remains nearly level, before beginning a steady rise with advancing age. Thus, in the later years, the risk of death is greater in each successive year of life. Such statements, which can be rapidly made from inspection of the hazard function, are not so easily extracted from the survival or death density functions themselves. Thus, it is often informative to examine the hazard function when time to response data are being analyzed.

Another important complication in survival analysis is the presence of censored observations. Frequently, analysis precedes the failure of all subjects, so that complete information is unavailable. In preclinical experiments, single-point right-hand censoring occurs, in that the study is terminated after a fixed length of observation for all subjects. In clinical experiments the censoring is progressive, as staggered entry into the trial causes varying lengths of follow-up or withdrawals.

Censored observations supply information only while they are
under observation and contribute to the likelihood function
through the survivorship function rather than through the death
density function.

3.2 REGRESSION METHODS IN SURVIVAL ANALYSIS

In an approach not immediately developed for application to
dose optimization, Feigl and Zelen [7] suggest a regression
method for relating concomitant information to the survival
times of patients with cancer. In this approach it is assumed
that the underlying survival distribution for the ith patient
is exponential with parameter λ_i. By expressing λ_i as a function of the concomitant variable x, the survival distribution
is made to depend upon the value of the concomitant variable
x_i for the ith patient. Feigl and Zelen consider the case
where λ_i is expressed as a linear function of x_i.

Specifically, let t_1, t_2, ..., t_n be a sample of n independent survival times, where the survival time for the ith
patient has the exponential probability density function

$$f_i(t) = \lambda_i \exp(-\lambda_i t) \qquad \text{for } t \geq 0$$
$$= 0 \qquad \text{for } t < 0$$

In addition, let x_1, x_2, ..., x_n be observed values of an important covariate with prognostic significance, e.g., performance status, weight loss, age, etc. Further, let it be
related to the survival times in such a manner that the mean
survival time for the ith patient, $E(t_i)$, is given by

$$E(t_i) = \frac{1}{\lambda_i} = \beta_0 + \beta_1 x_1$$

Under this model, the likelihood of the sample of n survival
times becomes

$$L = \prod_{i=1}^{n} f_i(t)$$

$$= \prod_{i=1}^{n} (\beta_0 + \beta_1 x_i)^{-1} \left\{ \exp\left[-\sum_{i=1}^{n} (\beta_0 + \beta_1 x_i)^{-1} t_i \right] \right\}$$

As a result, the log likelihood function is

$$\ln L = -\sum_{i=1}^{n} \ln(\beta_0 + \beta_1 x_i) - \sum_{i=1}^{n} (\beta_0 + \beta_1 x_i)^{-1} t_i$$

The maximum-likelihood estimators of β_0 and β_1 can be found by simultaneously solving

$$\frac{\partial(\ln L)}{\partial \beta_0} = -\sum_{i=1}^{n} (\beta_0 + \beta_1 x_i)^{-1} + \sum_{i=1}^{n} (\beta_0 + \beta_1 x_i)^{-2} t_i = 0$$

$$\frac{\partial(\ln L)}{\partial \beta_1} = -\sum_{i=1}^{n} (\beta_0 + \beta_1 x_i)^{-1} x_i + \sum_{i=1}^{n} (\beta_0 + \beta_1 x_i)^{-2} x_i t_i = 0$$

Notice that the equations are nonlinear in β_0 and β_1; consequently, iterative methods are required to obtain a solution.

The probability of the ith patient surviving at least to time t, $S_i(t)$, is given by

$$S_i(t) = \int_{t}^{\infty} f_i(u)\, du$$

$$= \exp(-\lambda_i t)$$

$$= \exp[-(\beta_0 + \beta_1 x)^{-1} t]$$

which can be estimated by

$$S_i(t) = \exp[-(\hat{\beta}_0 + \hat{\beta}_1 x)^{-1} t]$$

Using this expression, it is possible to test the adequacy of the model by comparing the observed numbers of patients dying in certain time intervals to the expected number of deaths in those intervals as a result of the model formulation. Let $t_i(p)$ be the point on the estimated survival distribution $S_i(t)$ of the patient with concomitant variate value x_i, for which the probability of survival is p, i.e.,

$$\hat{S}_i(t_i(p)) = \exp[-(\hat{\beta}_0 + \hat{\beta}_1 x_i)^{-1} t_i(p)]$$
$$= p$$

If p is chosen to be the quartile probabilities, the quartile intervals $[0, t_i(0.25)]$, $[t_i(0.25), t_i(0.50)]$, $[t_i(0.50), t_i(0.75)]$, $[t_i(0.75), \infty]$ for the ith patient (i = 1, 2, ..., n) can be determined. By construction, the probability for the ith patient to fail in any one of these intervals is 0.25. As a result, when the model provides a good fit to the data one-quarter of the patients should be expected to die in each of the four intervals. Departures from this expectation can be determined through use of the χ^2 test. It should be noted in testing for the goodness of fit of the model that the choice of fractile is arbitrary but should be governed by the concern that the expected number of failures per interval should be large enough to insure the validity of the χ^2 test.

Note that the above development has dealt with the situation of complete information on the failure of all subjects. The method has been extended by Zippin and Armitage [17] so that data sets which include censored observations can be analyzed.

While neither Feigl and Zelen nor Zippin and Armitage employed levels of treatment as concomitant variables, it is clear that their method can be used to relate survival experience to treatment levels. Once this has been accomplished it is then possible to obtain estimates of treatment levels associated with maximum average survival time and to estimate the survival distribution.

Glasser [8] suggested another approach for relating concomitant information to the survival experience of different
groups of individuals. In this development, which assumes an
underlying exponential distribution, the parameter for the ith
individual in the jth group, λ_{ij}, is written as

$$\lambda_{ij} = \lambda_j \exp(\beta x_{ij})$$

where x_{ij} is the value of the covariate for that individual.
From this formulation the maximum-likelihood estimators of λ_j
and β are developed along with the estimates of the corresponding survival distributions. In conclusion, Glasser notes that
the model can be extended to the situation with multiple covariates by writing

$$\lambda_{ij} = \lambda_j \exp(\beta_1 x_{1ij} + \beta_2 x_{2ij} + \cdots + \beta_k x_{kij})$$

It is finally noted that some of the x's can be functions of
the others, e.g., $x_{2ij} = x_{1ij}^2$.

Yet another method for relating response time data to
levels of concomitant variables via a regression analysis was
proposed by Myers, Hankey, and Mantel [13]. By assuming an
underlying exponential failure-time distribution, the probability of the ith individual surviving a time interval of unit
length is $Q_1 = \exp(-\lambda_i)$. Let T_i represent those of several
ordered and unit-length time intervals in which the ith subject responded or failed. Then the likelihood of a sample of
N individuals for which T_i, i = 1, 2, ..., N, are recorded
becomes

$$L = \prod_{i=1}^{N} Q_i^{T_i - 1} (1 - Q_i)$$

since for a person to respond in a given interval T, that individual must be a nonresponder in the T - 1 preceding intervals. Notice that L can be rewritten as

$$L = \prod_{i=1}^{N} Q_i^{T_i} \left(\frac{1 - Q_i}{Q_i} \right)^{Z_i}$$

where Z_i equals 1 if the ith individual is a responder and equals 0 otherwise.

The authors note that the logistic function has been widely used to relate the dependence of a response/no-response variable Y to a univariate or a multivariate regressor variable X. A general form of the function is given by

$$P(Y_i = \text{response} \mid X = X_i) = \{1 + \exp[-f(X_i; \underline{\beta})]\}^{-1}$$

or

$$P(Y_i = \text{no response} \mid X = X_i) = \exp[-f(X_i; \underline{\beta})]$$
$$\times \{1 + \exp[-f(X_i; \underline{\beta})]\}^{-1}$$

in which Y_i is the value of the response variable for the ith subject with regressor variable X_i and $f(X_i; \beta)$ is an arbitrary real-valued function of X_i and the parameter vector $\underline{\beta}$. A property of the logistic function is

$$\ell n \left(\frac{P(Y_i = \text{response} \mid X = X_i)}{P(Y_i = \text{no response} \mid X = X_i)} \right) = f(X_i; \underline{\beta})$$

By taking advantage of this property and assuming that

$$f(x_i; \beta) = \sum_{j=0}^{r} \beta_j x_{ji}$$

where the x_{ji} (j = 0, 1, ..., r) are the concomitant variable values for the ith individual, such that $x_{0i} = 1$ for each individual, we have

$$\ell n \left(\frac{P(Y_i = \text{response} \mid x = x_i)}{P(Y_i = \text{no response} \mid x = x_i)} \right) = \ell n \left(\frac{1 - Q_i}{Q_i} \right) = \sum_{j=0}^{r} \beta_j x_{ji}$$

As a result, the likelihood function can be rewritten as

$$L = \prod_{i=1}^{N} Q_i^{T_i} \left[\exp\left(\sum_{j=0}^{r} \beta_j x_{ji} \right) \right]^{Z_i}$$

with

$$Q_i = \left[1 + \exp\left(\sum_{j=0}^{r} \beta_j x_{ji} \right) \right]^{-1}$$

and

$$\lambda_i = \ln\left[1 + \exp\left(\sum_{j=0}^{r} \beta_j x_{ji} \right) \right]$$

Iterative methods are required to obtain the solutions to the likelihood equations. The authors note that the model is not time-scale invariant and discuss how the addition of a parameter which essentially defines what constitutes a time interval of observation can be used to avoid this problem. However, in the example that accompanies their work, it appears that the model's fit to the data is not dependent upon whether the additional parameter's value is fixed in advance or estimated from the data. The conclusion then is that for future applications, one might specify in advance the value to be used for the width of the time interval. When this is done the computational problems are simplified and, since there is one less variable, the confidence limits on the other parameters are narrower.

3.3 PROPORTIONAL HAZARD MODEL

In the previous section each of the methods discussed required an assumption about the parametric form of the survival distribution. In fact, all assumed, possibly for computational simplicity, a constant hazard function which results in an exponential survival distribution. Clearly, each approach could

be altered to consider more complicated hazard functions, but
in any case, some assumption as to the form of this function
must be made. Frequently, this form is unknown and it may not
always follow the well-established functional forms available.

Cox [3] initiated an important branch of survival analysis
with a regression model that permits nonparametric assessment
of the relationships among hazard functions. Cox's hazard-
based model is such that the risk function for an individual
with concomitant vector $\underline{x}$ is the product of an underlying hazard function $\lambda_0(t)$ and its multiplier, a function of the concomitant information. He describes the relation as

$$\lambda(t) = \lambda_0(t) \exp(\underline{x}'\underline{\beta})$$

where $\underline{x}$ is the concomitant information and $\underline{\beta}$ parameterizes the
model. Information on the effect of the concomitant data is
included in $\exp(\underline{x}'\underline{\beta})$ and since $\lambda(t)/\lambda_0(t) = \exp(\underline{x}'\underline{\beta})$, this
quantity is defined to be the relative hazard function.

If a parametric form for $\lambda_0(t)$ is assumed, a full likelihood function can be derived by noting the relationship between
the hazard and death density functions. In fact, if $\lambda_0(t)$ is
chosen to be constant, the model discussed by Glasser [8]
results.

Instead, Cox lets $\lambda_0(t)$ be an arbitrary function. He then
makes a conditional argument in developing what he terms a
conditional likelihood function. Given that a death occurs at
time t_j, the probability that it was individual i is the ratio
of $\lambda_i(t)$ to $\Sigma_{s \in R(t_j)} \lambda_s(t)$, where $R(t_j)$, the risk set, is the
set of all subjects known to be alive just prior to t_j. Thus,

$$L_j = \frac{\lambda_0(t) \exp(\underline{x}_{\underline{i}}'\underline{\beta})}{\Sigma_{s \in R(t_j)} \lambda_0(t) \exp(\underline{x}_{\underline{s}}'\underline{\beta})} = \frac{\exp(\underline{x}_{\underline{i}}'\underline{\beta})}{\Sigma_{s \in R(t_j)} \exp(\underline{x}_{\underline{s}}'\underline{\beta})}$$

A likelihood function is developed as the product of factors of
this type for each death. If one considers a situation where

the concomitant information has no effect, i.e., $\underline{x}'_i\underline{\beta} = 0$ for each individual, the contribution to the likelihood at time j is

$$\frac{\exp(0)}{\Sigma_{s\epsilon R(t_j)}\;\exp(0)} = \frac{1}{n_j}$$

In other words, providing no effect of the covariates exists, the chance of an individual having failed at t_j is just the reciprocal of the number at risk, as each individual's risk is equally weighted. If covariates are important, each subject's risk will be defined by $\exp(\underline{x}'\underline{\beta})$ and the above equation for L_j can be seen to equal the ratio of the individual's score to the total score of all subjects on study at time t_j. Ordinarily, the parameters $\underline{\beta}$ will be unknown, and the method of maximum-likelihood estimation can be used to determine their estimates.

Providing $\underline{x}$ is independent of time, Cox's formulation is called the proportional hazard model. The relative hazard function $\exp(\underline{x}'\underline{\beta})$ is constant through time and the survival distributions for different $\underline{x}$ are related as powers of each other. That is,

$$S(t) = \exp\left[-\int_0^t \lambda_0(u)\;\exp(\underline{x}'\underline{\beta})\;du\right]$$
$$= (S_0(t))^{\exp(\underline{x}'\underline{\beta})}$$

Similarly, if $\lambda_i(t)$ is twice as great as $\lambda_k(t)$ at time t, the same relationship is required at all other time points. Thus, the ordering and the separation of treatment values are constant.

A real advantage of this approach is that inference can be restricted to the effect of concomitant information without knowledge of the form of the survival distribution. As the parametric form of the hazard function is often unknown, this is of substantial value. Further, one must appreciate that interest is usually centered on the covariates as opposed to

the underlying survival distribution. Thus, the model permits
an important relaxation of the necessity to specify a function
which is not of utmost interest.

Cox's likelihood function has been the cause of some theoretical concern. In their discussion Kalbfleisch and Prentice
[9] noted that the likelihood function is not a conditional
one. Later they (Kalbfleisch and Prentice [10]) developed the
likelihood based on the marginal distribution of the ranks of
the survival times. Cox's likelihood was shown to be a marginal likelihood but only under certain restrictions, including
the requirement that the covariates not be functions of time.
Cox [4] responded with the theory of partial likelihoods, of
which both marginal and conditional likelihoods are special
cases. He noted that the hazard function, a nuisance parameter
as regards the relationships among the $\underline{x}_i$, can be excluded from
the partial likelihood and that regular large-sample statistical properties apply.

A major problem in the application of the partial likelihood function to many experimental situations is the presence
of a considerable amount of grouped survival times. In murine
cancer chemotherapy experiments, mice similar with respect to
genetic strain, sex, and weight are injected with identical
tumor masses and subsequently treated. As survival is often
assessed daily, substantial numbers of recorded tied survival
times necessarily result. Tied times of death do not actually
occur with a continuous hazard function, but nominally tied
survival times in this type of experiment are unavoidable.

This grouping of survival times leads to practical diffi-
culties in the analysis. If survival times for only subjects
1 and 2 were tied, one could calculate the real probability as
the sum of the probabilities that subject 1 died first and
subject 2 second, plus the probability of the reverse order.
That is

$$P_{Real} = \frac{\exp(\underline{x}_1'\beta)}{\Sigma_{i\epsilon R(t_j)} \exp(\underline{x}_i'\beta)} \frac{\exp(\underline{x}_2'\beta)}{\Sigma_{i\epsilon R(t_j)} \exp(\underline{x}_i'\beta) - \exp(\underline{x}_1'\beta)}$$

$$+ \frac{\exp(\underline{x}_2'\beta)}{\Sigma_{i\epsilon R(t_j)} \exp(\underline{x}_i'\beta)} \frac{\exp(\underline{x}_1'\beta)}{\Sigma_{i\epsilon R(t_j)} \exp(\underline{x}_i'\beta) - \exp(\underline{x}_2'\beta)}$$

But the number of terms in P_{Real} is $m_j!$ if the number of ties is m_j. This would prove to be computationally cumbersome with increasingly grouped data. Cox developed a logistic model in discrete time and approximated the probability for the above example as the ratio of the product of relative hazards for units 1 and 2 divided by the sum of the product of the relative hazards for all possible sets of two subjects, i.e.,

$$P_{Cox} = \frac{\exp(\underline{x}_1'\beta) \exp(\underline{x}_2'\beta)}{\Sigma_{(i<k)\epsilon R(t_j)} \exp(\underline{x}_i'\beta) \exp(\underline{x}_k'\beta)}$$

Peto [16] and Breslow [1, 2] suggested an alternative, less cumbersome approximation

$$P_{P-B} = 2 \frac{\exp(\underline{x}_1'\beta)}{N\{[\Sigma_{i\epsilon R(t_j)} \exp(\underline{x}_i'\beta)]/N\}}$$

$$\times \frac{\exp(\underline{x}_2'\beta)}{(N-1)\{[\Sigma_{i\epsilon R(t_j)} \exp(\underline{x}_i'\beta)]/N\}}$$

where N is the number of subjects in the risk set. Here, addition of another tied survival point will cause a reduction in the denominator's next factor equal to the average relative hazard. Kalbfleisch and Prentice [10] have another solution for their likelihood, but it is more cumbersome than Peto's suggestion. Although other suggestions have been made--for example, Efron [6] developed a potentially more accurate approximation--no advantages to the latter methods have been demonstrated. Due to its computational speed, theoretical

appropriateness, and extensive use, the Peto-Breslow approach
for handling tied failure times will be employed to deal with
nominally tied survival times in the remainder of this text.

Consider now the estimation of $\underline{\beta}$ by the method of maximum
likelihood. Suppose that there are m_j deaths observed out of
a possible r_j subjects at risk of death on day j. Then the
partial likelihood as modified to deal with ties is

$$\prod_{j=1}^{K} \frac{\Pi_{i=1}^{m_j} \exp(\underline{x}'_{ij}\underline{\beta})}{\binom{r_j}{m_j}[\Sigma_{v \in R(t_j)} \exp(\underline{x}'_{v}\underline{\beta})/r_j]^{m_j}} \tag{3.7}$$

where $R(t_j)$, the risk set, is composed of all subjects at risk
of death at time t_j and K is the number of times at which failures occur. Further, the log likelihood ignoring terms not
involving $\underline{\beta}$ is

$$\ln L \propto \sum_{j=1}^{K} \left[\sum_{i=1}^{m_j} \underline{x}'_{ij}\underline{\beta} - m_j \ln \sum_{v \in R(t_j)} \exp(\underline{x}'_{v}\underline{\beta}) \right]$$

Iterative methods are required to obtain the resulting estimates. Pursuing the maximization often requires taking first
derivatives with respect to $\underline{\beta}_s$ (s = 1, 2, ..., p), where p is
the number of parameters in the model and second derivatives
with respect to $\underline{\beta}_s$ and $\underline{\beta}_t$ (s, t = 1, 2, ..., p), where $\underline{x}$ =
$(x_1, x_2, ..., x_p)$. The parameter estimates $\hat{\underline{\beta}}$ are the solution
to the p equations

$$\frac{\partial(\ln L)}{\partial \beta_s} = \sum_{j=1}^{k} \left[\sum_{i=1}^{m_j} x_{ijs} - \frac{m_j \Sigma_{v \in R(t_j)} x_{vs} \exp(\underline{x}'_{v}\underline{\beta})}{\Sigma_{v \in R(t_j)} \exp(\underline{x}'_{v}\underline{\beta})} \right] = 0 \tag{3.8}$$

where the second derivatives are

$$\frac{\partial^2 (\ell n\ L)}{\partial \beta_s\ \partial \beta_t} = \sum_{j=1}^{k} \left\{ - \frac{m_j}{\Sigma_{v \in R(t_j)}\ \exp(\underline{x}'_v\underline{\beta})^2} \right.$$

$$\times\ [\Sigma_{v \in R(t_j)}\ \exp(\underline{x}'\underline{\beta})\ \Sigma_{v \in R(t_j)} x_{vt} x_{vs}\ \exp(\underline{x}'\underline{\beta})$$

$$\left. -\ \Sigma_{v \in R(t_j)} x_{vt}\ \exp(\underline{x}'_v\underline{\beta})\ \Sigma_{v \in R(t_j)} x_{vs}\ \exp(\underline{x}'_v\underline{\beta})] \right\}$$

Maximum-likelihood estimation permits asymptotic tests for parameter and model significance. The likelihood-ratio criterion can be used to assess significance since twice the difference in log partial likelihood of the full model with $p + p_1$ parameters, less that of the p-parameter model, is distributed asymptotically as a $\chi^2_{p_1}$ random variable. A test of the hypothesis that $\underline{\beta} = 0$ effectively tests for model significance. Alternatively, the asymptotic normality of β can be used to test the hypothesis that $C\underline{\beta} = 0$, since $\hat{\underline{\beta}}'C'[C(-I^{-1})C']^{-1}C\hat{\underline{\beta}}$ is asymptotically distributed as χ_u^2 if C is full rank u which is less than or equal to the dimensionality of β and the iith element of I, Fisher's information matrix, is given by

$$\hat{I}_{ij} = \frac{\partial^2 (\ell n\ L)}{\partial \beta_i\ \partial \beta_j}$$

Peace and Flora [15], in a Monte Carlo study, have compared the properties of the test based on the likelihood-ratio criterion to those of the test based on the asymptotic normality of the maximum-likelihood estimators. For sample sizes considered, these authors were unable to show any clear superiority associated with either method.

The partial likelihood function can be used to test for equality of two survival distributions, by including a dummy variate x_1 equal to 0 or 1 and testing that $\beta_1 = 0$. This is asymptotically equivalent, in the absence of tied failure times, to the Mantel-Haenszel test. Further, the similarity of these

approaches in small-sample situations has been explored. It
is our intention here to employ the proportional hazard model
in response surface analysis of cancer combination chemotherapy.

For the analysis to successfully explore interrelation-
ships among the drugs and to successfully locate the optimum,
the fitted response model must approximate the true surface in
the region of the experiment. From empirical considerations,
it appears likely that for any instant in time t, the value of
the hazard function will decrease with increasing levels of
treatment until toxicity becomes important. From that point
in the treatment space on, the value of the hazard function is
likely to increase. As a result, $\underline{x}'\underline{\beta}$ may be chosen to be a
second-degree polynomial in the treatment variables. For ex-
ample, if a three-drug combination is being studied

$$\underline{x}'\underline{\beta} = \beta_1 x_1 + \beta_2 x_2 + \beta_3 x_3 + \beta_{11} x_1^2 + \beta_{22} x_2^2 + \beta_{33} x_3^2$$
$$+ \beta_{12} x_1 x_2 + \beta_{13} x_1 x_3 + \beta_{23} x_2 x_3$$

where x_i (i = 1, 2, 3) is a function of the dose of drug i.
Notice that no intercept term is included. Any constant or
function of time alone can be factored out of the relative
hazard function and associated with $\lambda_0(t)$.

After one estimates the model parameters it is possible
to obtain estimates of the treatment levels $\underline{x}$ which maximize
the probability of survival to time t. This is determined by

$$\max_{\underline{x}} S(t) = \max_{\underline{x}} \exp\left[-\int_0^t \lambda_0(u) \exp(\underline{x}'\underline{\beta}) \, du\right]$$

An estimate of this can be obtained by replacing the parameters
with their estimates and taking the logarithm, i.e.,

$$\max_{\underline{x}} \hat{S}(t) = \max_{\underline{x}}\left[- \exp(\underline{x}'\hat{\underline{\beta}}) \int_0^t \lambda_0(u) \, du\right]$$

which corresponds to min $\underline{x}'\hat{\underline{\beta}}$. With combinations containing
only a few drugs, this maximization is algebraically simple,
but often the stationary point found is outside the experimental region. To insure that the estimated optimal treatment is
obtained within the region of experimentation, it is usually
necessary to place constraints on the solution. The direct-
optimization procedure developed by Nelder and Mead [14] is
quite useful for this constrained optimization.

The relationships, if known, between the drugs in a combination contain information which can be used to advantage in
the development of better treatments. While the estimate of
the optimal treatment levels is valuable in its own right, it
indicates only where the hazard response surface is minimized.
Thus, it provides an estimate of the location of the minimum
which is a result of the relationships among the drugs, without
providing information concerning these relationships. Although
$\exp(\underline{x}'\beta)$ is not the estimated hazard function, it is proportional to it. Therefore contour plots of this quantity, the rela-
tive hazard function, provide a graphic representation of the
manner in which the hazard function is influenced by the relationships among the drugs in combination. The contours of constant response will be plotted as in the previous chapter so
that darker shading indicates improved treatment. With the
proportional hazards model improved treatment is associated
with lower values of the relative risk of failure.

Notice that the values of the relative hazard function are
scale dependent, as $\lambda_0(t)$ corresponds to that hazard function
with $\underline{x} = \underline{0}$. If uncentered drug dosages are used in the analysis and the treatments are effective, then $\exp(\underline{x}'\underline{\beta})$ will be
less than 1, unless $\underline{x}$ is a very toxic dose. If instead $\underline{x}$ is
scaled by dosages at the center of the experimental design, all
comparisons are made with respect to this point. Values of the
relative hazard both greater than and less than 1 would be

expected, unless the design center is also the optimum. In the
latter situation $\exp(\underline{x}'\underline{\beta}) > 1$ for every $\underline{x}$.

3.4 CONFIDENCE REGION FOR THE OPTIMAL TREATMENT COMBINATION

In the proportional hazards model the levels of treatment are
related to treatment outcome through the function $\underline{x}'\underline{\beta}$. When a
full quadratic is used, it is such that the expression for
$\partial\underline{x}'\underline{\beta}/\partial x_i$ (i = 1, 2, ..., k, where k is the number of drugs in
the combination), is identical to that found in the quadratic
logistic regression case. Thus, the development of the confidence region for the optimal treatment combination in the proportional hazard model parallels that given in Chap. 2 for the
logistic model.

3.5 EXAMPLES AND MODEL FIT

In Table 3.1 the results are given of an experiment testing the
effectiveness of cisplatin (DDP) and 5-fluorouracil (5-FU)
in combination as the treatment of P388 murine leukemia. Mice
were injected with 10^6 cells i.p. on day 0 and treated on day 7
with the dosage levels indicated in this table.

Upon estimating the parameters of the proportional hazard
model, one obtains the elements presented in Table 3.2, where
it is clear that significant effects, both beneficial and harmful, are associated with the dosages used in this experiment.
From the plot of the ℓn relative hazard function (Fig. 3.1)
toxicity associated with high dosages of either treatment is
visible. A clear synergy is evidenced by the closed elliptical
regions where the estimated optimal treatment combination is
found to be.

To assess model fit, one can examine the relationship between the observed and predicted average survival times. As
the model requires that all survival curves be powers of each

TABLE 3.1. *Survival and Treatment Data from Original 5-FU/DDP Experiment*

Treatment (mg/kg)		
5-FU	DDP	Survival times (days)
0.00	0.00	9,10(2)[a],11(5)
23.70	5.20	14(3),15(4),18
32.30	10.30	15,17(2),18(3),19(2)
32.30	2.60	13(7),14
64.60	13.80	13,15,16(2),18,19,20(2)
64.60	5.20	15,16,17(4),18(2)
64.60	1.90	12,13,14(3),15(2),16
129.00	10.30	14,15,16,17,18,19,20,21
129.00	2.60	14,16(4),17(2),18
172.00	5.20	18(4),19(3)
64.60	0.00	10,13(6),14
129.00	0.00	14,15(7)
215.00	0.00	15(2),16(6)
0.00	5.20	13(6),14(2)
0.00	10.30	10,14(2),15(4),17
0.00	17.20	13(2),14(3),15,16,18

[a]The number in parentheses indicates the number of deaths on that day.

other, only the values of the relative hazard and not the distributions themselves are needed to enable the ordering of the fitted average survival times. Correlating the ranks of the median survival times for each treatment group with the ranks of the estimated relative hazards, one obtains a measure of the model fit. Note that this is an assessment, much like the coefficient of determination R^2 from a standard regression analysis, that is basically explanatory. It does not assure one of the predictive capability of the model.

TABLE 3.2. Parameter Estimates, Tests of Significance, and Covariance Matrix for the Original 5-FU/DDP Experiment

Parameter	Maximum-likelihood estimate	Significance
β_1 (5-FU)	-0.05784058	$p < 0.0001$
β_2 (DDP)	-0.85198541	$p < 0.0001$
β_{11}	0.00015744	$p < 0.0001$
β_{22}	0.03282069	$p < 0.0001$
β_{12}	0.00247116	$p = 0.0002$

$$
\text{var } \hat{\underline{\beta}} = \begin{bmatrix}
0.908207 \times 10^{-4} & 0.8469497 \times 10^{-3} & -0.314451 \times 10^{-6} & -0.31657 \times 10^{-4} & -0.52826 \times 10^{-5} \\
0.8469497 \times 10^{-3} & 0.1501261 \times 10^{-1} & -0.24274 \times 10^{-5} & -0.655114 \times 10^{-3} & -0.672468 \times 10^{-5} \\
-0.314451 \times 10^{-6} & -0.24274 \times 10^{-5} & 0.118626 \times 10^{-8} & 0.88036 \times 10^{-7} & 0.165756 \times 10^{-7} \\
-0.31657 \times 10^{-4} & -0.655114 \times 10^{-3} & 0.88036 \times 10^{-7} & 0.3087753 \times 10^{-4} & 0.27064 \times 10^{-5} \\
-0.52826 \times 10^{-5} & -0.672468 \times 10^{-5} & 0.165756 \times 10^{-7} & 0.27064 \times 10^{-5} & 0.454197 \times 10^{-6}
\end{bmatrix}
$$

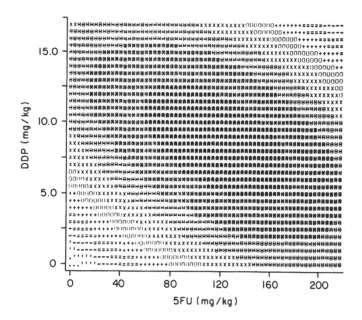

FIGURE 3.1. *Plot of contours of constant ℓn relative hazard from the original 5-FU/DDP experiment. The range of estimated ℓn relative hazard associated with each symbol is as follows:*

· · · · · ·	0.000 to -0.390	++++++	-2.732 to -3.513
' ' ' ' ' '	-0.390 to -1.171	000000	-3.513 to -4.293
– – –	-1.171 to -1.951	XXXXXX	-4.293 to -5.074
======	-1.951 to -2.732	ΘΘΘΘΘΘ	-2.734 to -3.300

℞℞℞℞℞℞	-5.854 to -6.635
ΘΘΘΘΘΘ	-6.635 to -7.025

The median survival time and the value of the relative hazard function for each of the treatment groups are given in Table 3.3. From the ranks of these the Spearman correlation coefficient is calculated to be -0.9451, which is significantly different from 0 (p = 0.0001). Because of the explanatory nature of this statistic, a minimal requirement for placing confidence in further detailed analyses of the estimated response function is that the magnitude of the correlation is large.

TABLE 3.3. Median Survival Times and Values of
the Relative Hazard Function for Treatment Groups
in the Original 5-FU/DDP Experiment

Treatment (mg/kg)		Relative hazard	Median survival (days)
5-FU	DDP		
0.00	0.00	1.00000	11.0
23.70	5.20	0.01088	15.0
32.30	10.30	0.00208	18.0
32.30	2.60	0.03051	13.0
64.60	13.80	0.00169	17.0
64.60	5.20	0.00305	17.0
64.60	1.90	0.01389	14.0
129.00	10.30	0.00106	17.5
129.00	2.60	0.00246	16.0
172.00	5.20	0.00133	18.0
64.60	0.00	0.04598	13.0
129.00	0.00	0.00790	15.0
215.00	0.00	0.00575	16.0
0.00	5.20	0.02893	13.0
0.00	10.30	0.00502	15.0
0.00	17.20	0.00712	14.0

Other procedures to examine fit require the estimation of
the hazard function or of the survival distribution. Kaplan
and Meier [11] discuss the estimation of these functions when
only a single distribution is considered. They develop a maximum-likelihood estimate under the class of admissible distributions, but their estimate of the hazard function at time j,
$\hat{\lambda}_j(t) = \delta_j/n_j$, where n_j equals the size of the risk set at time
t_j and δ_j equals the number of failures at t_j, is a discrete
function in discontinuous time having mass only at time points
where failures occur. Thus, the hazard estimate is just the

observed probability of failures at t_j. Their estimate of the
survival distribution is then

$$\hat{S}(t) = \prod_{j=1}^{K} \left(1 - \frac{\delta_j}{n_j}\right)$$

where failures occur at k distinct time points.

Risk, though, is commonly perceived to be a continuous
function, with hazard associated with every instant of time.
An estimate, unlike the above, consistent with this perception
is desirable, and it further simplifies the estimation of survival distributions when multiple treatment groups are considered. Breslow [2] suggests that within intervals between
failure times the hazard be estimated by a constant. Thus, in
the interval (t_{j-1}, t_j)

$$\hat{\lambda}_{j-1,j}(t) = \frac{\delta_j}{(t_j - t_{j-1})n_j}$$

so that the point mass risk of Kaplan and Meier has been evenly
spread over the interval, and the hazard function is estimated
by a step function with discontinuities at failure times.

For applications with more than a single survival distribution, such as the combination experiments, one can replace
δ_j and n_j with their corresponding scores from the proportional
hazard model. One can estimate the underlying hazard for $\underline{x} = \underline{0}$
with parameter estimates $\hat{\underline{\beta}}$ as

$$\hat{\lambda}_{0,j-1,j}(t) = \frac{\Sigma_{j=1}^{m_j} \exp(\underline{0}'\hat{\underline{\beta}})}{(t_j - t_{j-1}) \Sigma_{s \in R(t_j)} \exp(\underline{x}_s'\hat{\underline{\beta}})}$$

$$= \frac{m_j}{(t_j - t_{j-1}) \Sigma_{s \in R(t_j)} \exp(\underline{x}_s'\hat{\underline{\beta}})}$$

The survival distribution for any treated group can be estimated as

$$\hat{S}(t) = \exp\left[-\int_0^t \exp(\underline{x}'\hat{\underline{\beta}}) \ \hat{\lambda}_0(u) \ du\right] \qquad (3.9)$$

Note, further, that if the relative hazard is a function of time, $\exp[g(x, t)]$, as in the succeeding chapter, the hazard function can be estimated as

$$\hat{\lambda}_{0,j-1,j}(t) = \frac{m_j}{\int_{t_{j-1}}^{t_j} \Sigma_{s\in R(t_j)} \ \exp[g(\underline{x}, u)] \ du} \qquad (3.10)$$

Observed and fitted survival distributions can be examined to assess their closeness by evaluating Eq. (3.9) for each treatment combination. Although overall tests for fit can be developed rather readily, as, for example, the χ^2 test used by Feigl and Zelen [7], for our application it is important to determine fit in each region of the experiment. Here, as with the logistic regression approach, small sample sizes for each of the experimental groups make such statistical determinations difficult.

Another value of estimating the hazard function is in the examination of fit via the methods of residual analysis following Kay [12] and Cox and Snell [5]. Effectively, residuals ε_i are defined as

$$\varepsilon_i = \int_0^{t_i} \lambda_0(u) \ \exp(\underline{x}_i'\underline{\beta}) \ du$$

and substituting appropriate function estimates and survival times t_i yields the crude residuals. Residual estimates for censored survival times are always underestimates of the residual if the time of each were known. Kay proposes assuming an underlying unit-exponential error distribution. Thus, the crude residuals should behave as a censored sample from a unit exponential. Under this assumption, estimating the cumulative hazard distribution of the residuals will yield a line of unit slope if the fit is adequate.

For the experiment under consideration, Fig. 3.2 is a plot of the cumulative hazard function for the crude residuals. The fit appears to be adequate. Such a plot is often more valuable when several models are used, so that comparative fit can be examined.

The estimated optimal treatment combination is 116.4 mg/kg of 5-FU and 8.6 mg/kg of DDP. The estimated 95% confidence region about the optimal combination is given in Fig. 3.3. Unlike the confidence region given in Fig. 2.4, this region is closed. Indeed, the confidence region is smaller than the region of lowest relative hazard given in Fig. 3.1. While such a comparison is dependent on the scale used to describe the hazard contours, it is interesting to note that the orientation of the confidence region differs from that of the contours of constant response--a difference which is independent of the scale used.

As this analysis indicates that certain combinations of drug levels are superior to the single-drug optima, the combination was repeated in the L1210 tumor system with day-3 treatment.

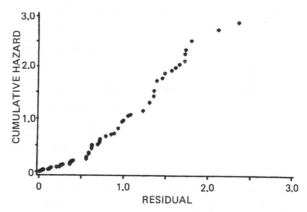

FIGURE 3.2. *Plot of cumulative hazard function for crude residuals from original 5-FU/DDP experiment.*

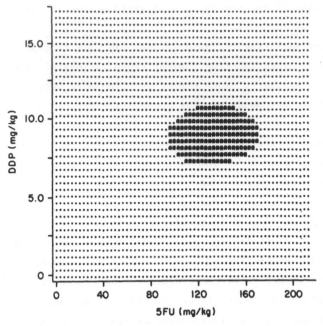

FIGURE 3.3. *Confidence region (95%) about optimal treatment
levels from original 5-FU/DDP experiment. Dosage levels within
the confidence region are indicated by the dark symbol.*

The design, a central composite with additional single-drug
controls, was augmented by four treatment groups selected
through considering the optimal region of the previous experiment. These four treatments are the last four listed in Table
3.4, which contains a summary of the experiment. Notice that
in three of the four treatments, the survival experience was
quite good, with 50% survivors in each. Of the 19 long-term
survivors, 12 are from these groups. When analyzed, the parameter estimates in Table 3.5 are obtained, where again parameter
significance is clearly established. Fit appears to be adequate with a Spearman rank-order correlation between the estimated relative hazard and median survival time of -0.84946
($p = 0.0001$). Marked similarity in the relative hazard

TABLE 3.4. *Treatment and Survival Data from Replicate 5-FU/DDP Experiment*

Treatment (mg/kg)		
5-FU	DDP	Survival times (days)
0.00	0.00	8(8)[a]
47.90	8.20	16(2),17,18(2),22(3)
65.30	16.30	10(2),20,24,26,112[+](3)
65.30	4.10	14,16(2),17,18,19,21
131.00	21.80	8,9(3),10(2),11,112[+]
131.00	8.20	10,12,17,18,26,29,112[+](2)
131.00	3.00	17,18,19(4),20(2)
261.00	16.30	9(4),10(2),12(2)
261.00	4.10	14,17,18,21,22,24,25,26
348.00	8.20	12(2),22(2),24(2),35,112[+]
47.90	0.00	10(2),12(6)
131.00	0.00	13(3),14(3),16(2)
348.00	0.00	9(2),10(4),12(2)
0.00	3.00	10(3),12(5)
0.00	8.20	12,13(3),14(3),16
0.00	21.80	8(2),9,13,17,21,24,25
152.00	13.60	9,18,21,61,112[+](4)
174.00	10.90	10,29,49,61,112[+](4)
196.00	8.20	10,22,25,65,112[+](4)
218.00	5.44	14,17,21(2),22,24,27,30

[a]The number in parentheses indicates the number of deaths on that day.

[+]Censored observation.

functions for the two experiments can be observed with the aid of Fig. 3.4. The optimal treatment levels estimated from the second experiment are 148.5 mg/kg of 5-FU and 11.1 mg/kg of DDP. The height of the surfaces indicates that in the L1210 experiment

TABLE 3.5. *Parameter Estimates, Tests of Significance, and Covariance Matrix for the Replicate 5-FU/DDP Experiment*

Parameter	Maximum-likelihood estimate	Significance
β_1(5-FU)	-0.02040651	$p < 0.0001$
β_2(DDP)	-0.47423867	$p < 0.0001$
β_{11}	0.00004221	$p < 0.0001$
β_{22}	0.01661461	$p < 0.0001$
β_{12}	0.00070849	$p < 0.0001$

$$\text{var } \hat{\underline{\beta}} = \begin{bmatrix} 0.1032374 \times 10^{-4} & 0.5145512 \times 10^{-4} & -0.218294 \times 10^{-7} & -0.902701 \times 10^{-6} & -0.291954 \times 10^{-6} \\ 0.5145512 \times 10^{-4} & 0.3418756 \times 10^{-2} & -0.723809 \times 10^{-7} & -0.126626 \times 10^{-3} & -0.55964 \times 10^{-5} \\ -0.218294 \times 10^{-7} & -0.723809 \times 10^{-7} & 0.567905 \times 10^{-10} & 0.15117 \times 10^{-8} & 0.287707 \times 10^{-9} \\ -0.902701 \times 10^{-6} & -0.126626 \times 10^{-3} & 0.15117 \times 10^{-8} & 0.524774 \times 10^{-5} & 0.150229 \times 10^{-6} \\ -0.291954 \times 10^{-6} & -0.55964 \times 10^{-5} & 0.287707 \times 10^{-9} & 0.150229 \times 10^{-6} & 0.29444 \times 10^{-7} \end{bmatrix}$$

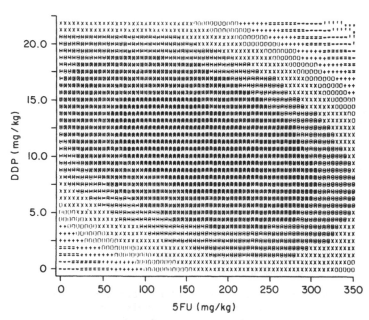

FIGURE 3.4. *Plot of contour of constant relative hazard from second 5-FU/DDP experiment.*

・・・・・・	0.943 to 0.660	++++++	-1.037 to -1.602
''''''	0.660 to 0.095	000000	-1.602 to -2.168
------	0.095 to -0.471	XXXXXX	-2.168 to -2.734
======	-0.471 to -1.037	ΘΘΘΘΘΘ	-2.734 to -3.300

៙៙៙៙៙៙	-3.300 to -3.865
⊕⊕⊕⊕⊕⊕	-3.865 to -4.148

a more substantial reduction of the underlying hazard results. Notice that having smaller relative hazard values does not indicate that the survival experience is better unless the underlying hazard function is the same. The confidence region about the optimal combination is given in Fig. 3.5.

Consider now the study of a three-drug combination using a proportional hazards model. The doses and resulting survival times from an experiment testing the combination of cyclophosphamide (CTX), doxorubicin (ADR), and 5-fluorouracil (5-FU) are included in Table 3.6, along with summary survival information.

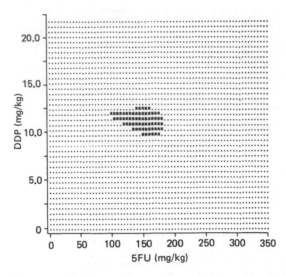

FIGURE 3.5. Confidence region about optimal treatment levels from second 5-FU/DDP experiment. Dosage levels within the confidence region are indicated by the dark symbol.

The 199 B6D2F$_1$ female mice were inoculated interperitoneally with 10^6 P388 leukemia cells on day 0 and divided into 24 groups of eight animals and 1 group of seven animals. Treatment occurred on day 7 with the doses indicated in the table. Consistent with previous approaches, a model quadratic in each of the drugs with all two-drug interactions included was used. Additionally, since one might want to add a term to indicate the simultaneous effects of the three drugs, both the 9-parameter and a 10-parameter model including a three drug interaction term were fitted. Of immediate interest is the test for significance of the three-factor interaction. The likelihood-ratio test for this parameter generates a test statistic with a value of 13.18 with an associated p value of 0.0003. This result suggests that the 10-parameter model may more appropriately represent the study results. In Table 3.7 the parameter estimates, their standard errors, and significance based on

TABLE 3.6. *Treatment and Survival Data from CTX/ADR/5-FU Experiment*

Treatment (mg/kg)			
CTX	ADR	5-FU	Survival times (days)
0.00	0.00	0.00	$9(7)^a,12$
36.80	0.74	18.40	19(2),21(2),22,25,26
230.00	0.74	18.40	$14,28(2),30,35,45,82^+(2)$
36.80	4.60	18.40	$9,23(2),25,38(2),82^+(2)$
36.80	0.74	115.00	9,19(2),21(3),23,24
230.00	4.60	18.40	$37,68,82^+(6)$
230.00	0.74	115.00	15,30(3),32,33,37,48
36.80	4.60	115.00	9,17,21,22,24(3),25
230.00	4.60	115.00	12,14(6),15
414.00	1.84	46.00	8(2),9(5),10
18.40	1.84	46.00	8,11,19(4),22,27
92.00	8.28	46.00	9,28,30,31(2),32(2),35
92.00	0.37	46.00	11,22(2),25(2),26,27,30
92.00	1.84	207.00	8,15,16,19,25(2),27,30
92.00	1.84	9.20	9,25,28(2),33(2),35,81
92.00	1.84	46.00	9,23,25(2),26,27,30,33
92.00	0.00	0.00	$9(2),12,23(2),25,26,82^+$
230.00	0.00	0.00	$30(2),34,35,37,38,40,82^+$
414.00	0.00	0.00	8(2),9(2),10,12,13,17
0.00	1.84	0.00	8,9(2),10(4),11
0.00	4.60	0.00	9,10(3),12,13,14(2)
0.00	8.28	0.00	9,10(4),14,23,30
0.00	0.00	46.00	8,10,11(2),13(2),14,15
0.00	0.00	115.00	10,13(2),14(4),15
0.00	0.00	207.00	10,13,14(4),15,21

[a]The number in parentheses indicates the number of deaths on that day.
[+]Censored observation.

TABLE 3.7. *Parameter Estimates, Standard Deviations, and Significance for the CTX/ADR/5-FU Experiment*

Parameter	Maximum-likelihood estimate	Standard deviation	Significance
β_1 (CTX)	-0.04080078	0.00373098	p < 0.0001
β_2 (ADR)	-0.54502810	0.13198516	p < 0.0001
β_3 (5-FU)	-0.01198830	0.00542245	p = 0.0270
β_{11}	0.00009676	0.00000838	p < 0.0001
β_{22}	0.03661546	0.01410859	p = 0.0095
β_{33}	0.00002473	0.00002260	p = 0.2737
β_{12}	-0.0005187	0.00063369	p = 0.4128
β_{13}	0.00004953	0.00002082	p = 0.0167
β_{23}	0.00171097	0.00107307	p = 0.1108
β_{123}	0.00003410	0.00000902	p = 0.0003

individual asymptotic normal theory tests are listed. Note that each of the linear and quadratic terms, with the exception of the quadratic 5-FU parameter, is individually significant. That the term in the model which accounts for 5-FU toxicity is not statistically significant is not surprising, as the doses of 5-FU used are sublethal. Since the three-drug interaction is significant, it follows that the two-drug interactions change with changing levels of the third drug. Note, though, that the interactions of CTX with 5-FU and ADR with 5-FU are deleterious no matter what the level of the other drugs and that the deleterious effect of the interaction increases with the level of the third drug. On the other hand, in the absence of 5-FU, the interaction between CTX and ADR is not harmful.

Continuing with the analysis, model fit, as measured by the Spearman correlation of rankings of predicted hazard and observed median survival, is adequate, with a correlation coefficient of -0.9443 (p = 0.0001). The dose response surface

of a three-drug combination is a four-dimensional figure. As
such, it cannot be displayed graphically. However, when one
of the drugs is considered at a fixed dosage level, it is possible to present the contours of constant response of the relationship between the other two drugs. Thus, by considering
several dosage levels of the fixed drug it is possible to gain
an appreciation of the underlying dose response surface. The
plots of the ℓn relative hazard function cross-sections for
fixed values of the third drug are displayed in Fig. 3.6. Examination of this figure indicates a decreasing effectiveness
of the CTX/ADR combination as the dosage of 5-FU increases.
Thus, the beneficial effects of 5-FU are overridden by the
toxic interactions with the other drugs. The plots of 5-FU
and CTX as well as 5-FU and ADR all indicate that 5-FU is relatively unimportant in the dose regions explored. Optimization
yields an estimate of the optimal treatment as 207.24 mg/kg of
CTX, 7.11 mg/kg of ADR, and 15.00 mg/kg of 5-FU. Note that
this result is consistent with the observation that the 12
animals alive on day 82 received minimal doses of 5-FU. As a
result of the analysis, a CTX/ADR synergy is evident, with no
added value associated with the inclusion of 5-FU.

Such straightforward results are not always the case.
Survival summaries of a similar experiment using vinblastine
(VLB), cisplatin (DDP), and bleomycin (BLM) in the treatment
of P388 leukemia are listed in Table 3.8. Again, the three-way
interaction term was significant, χ_1^2 = 6.54, p = 0.011. The
parameter estimates, their standard errors, and their significance are listed in Table 3.9. The Spearman rank-order correlation coefficient was calculated to be -0.5608 (p = 0.0036).
Note that both the linear and the quadratic terms for BLM are
positive and nearly significant. Thus, little or no treatment
advantage is associated with this drug alone. In addition,
the VLB/DDP interaction is significant and harmful, no matter

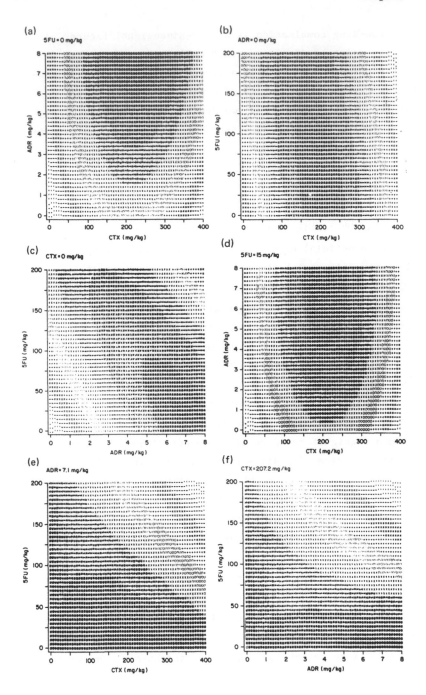

what the dose of BLM. Finally, the significant beneficial VLB/BLM interaction suggests that the latter drug may have some usefulness in combination. From the plots of the ℓn relative hazard function in Fig. 3.7, one can observe that BLM is an effective agent when a moderate dose of VLB is present, but not in the absence of VLB. Further, the drugs interact in such a manner as to suggest the use of low doses of DDP and high doses of BLM and VLB or low doses of VLB with high doses of DDP and BLM to achieve essentially similar effects. Obviously, replication of this experiment would be required to help clarify the latter point.

FIGURE 3.6. *Plots of contours of constant relative hazard from the CTX/ADR/5-FU experiment. Plots a, b, and c are made up of contours of the three possible two-drug combinations when the third drug is given at a zero level. Plots d, e, and f are made up of contours of the three possible two-drug combinations when the third drug is given at its estimated optimal level. The shadings for each panel have a different meaning. The two darkest areas, which constitute the region of interest, have values of -6.03 to -6.83 and -6.83 to -7.23, -3.34 to -4.00 and -4.00 to -4.33, -1.69 to -1.92 and -1.92 to -2.03, respectively, for the top three panels.*

TABLE 3.8.   *Treatment and Survival Data from*
VLB/DDP/BLM Experiment

Treatment (mg/kg)			
VLB	DDP	BLM	Survival times (days)
0.00	0.00	0.00	$9(3)^a$,10(2),11
0.89	1.78	2.66	13(2),14,15(2),26
5.55	1.78	2.66	21,23,27,28,32,35
0.89	11.10	2.66	12,13,26,35(2),38
0.89	1.78	16.60	14(2),15,17,19,27
5.55	11.10	2.66	9,11(2),12(2),14
5.55	1.78	16.60	20,22,24,27,35,38
0.89	11.10	16.60	11,14,23,24,26(2)
5.55	11.10	16.60	11(4),12,31
10.00	4.44	6.66	$11(2),13,31,38,300^+$
0.44	4.44	6.66	13,17,20(2),23,33
2.22	20.00	6.66	$11(2),12(2),14,300^+$
2.22	0.89	6.66	14(2),15,17,27(2)
2.22	4.44	30.00	$27,29,31(3),300^+$
2.22	4.44	1.33	20,21,22,27,29,35
2.22	4.44	6.66	$17,22,23(2),26,300^+$
2.22	0.00	0.00	11,12(2),14,15,26
5.55	0.00	0.00	14,15,17(3),20
10.00	0.00	0.00	9,13(2),17,19(2)
0.00	4.44	0.00	13,15,17,19(2),20
0.00	11.10	0.00	12,22,23,28(2),35
0.00	20.00	0.00	12,13(3),15,26
0.00	0.00	6.66	9(3),10(3)
0.00	0.00	16.60	9(2),10(4)
0.00	0.00	30.00	9(3),10,11(2)

[a]The number in parentheses indicates the number
of deaths on that day.

[+]Censored observation.

TABLE 3.9. *Parameter Estimates, Standard Deviations, and Significance for the VLB/DDP/BLM Experiment*

Parameter	Maximum-likelihood estimate	Standard deviation	Significance
β_1 (VLB)	-0.56057622	0.13606695	$p < 0.0001$
β_2 (DDP)	-0.38327009	0.06881985	$p < 0.0001$
β_3 (BLM)	0.01084254	0.04098849	$p = 0.7914$
β_{11}	0.04104696	0.01163499	$p = 0.0004$
β_{22}	0.01477855	0.00296051	$p < 0.0001$
β_{33}	0.00027762	0.00121238	$p = 0.8189$
β_{12}	0.03059901	0.01347633	$p = 0.0232$
β_{13}	-0.02350853	0.00816637	$p = 0.0040$
β_{23}	-0.00509627	0.00407723	$p = 0.2113$
β_{123}	0.00357950	0.00130303	$p = 0.0069$

Panel 1

```
······  -2.86 to -2.55      ++++++  -0.681 to -0.057
''''''  -2.55 to -1.93      000000  -0.057 to 0.567
------  -0.93 to -1.30      XXXXXX  0.567 to 1.191
======  -1.30 to -0.681     ΘΘΘΘΘΘ  1.191 to 1.815

                    ⍟⍟⍟⍟⍟⍟  1.815 to 2.439
                    ⊕⊕⊕⊕⊕⊕  2.439 to 2.751
```

Panel 2

```
······  -0.575 to -0.100    ++++++  2.751 to 3.702
''''''  -0.100 to 0.850     000000  3.702 to 4.652
------  0.850 to 1.801      XXXXXX  4.652 to 5.602
======  1.801 to 2.751      ΘΘΘΘΘΘ  5.602 to 6.553

                    ⍟⍟⍟⍟⍟⍟  6.553 to 7.503
                    ⊕⊕⊕⊕⊕⊕  7.503 to 7.978
```

Panel 3

```
······  -0.575 to -0.305    ++++++  1.316 to 1.856
''''''  -0.305 to 0.235     000000  1.856 to 2.397
------  0.235 to 0.776      XXXXXX  2.397 to 2.937
======  0.776 to 1.316      ΘΘΘΘΘΘ  2.937 to 3.477

                    ⍟⍟⍟⍟⍟⍟  3.477 to 4.018
                    ⊕⊕⊕⊕⊕⊕  4.018 to 4.288
```

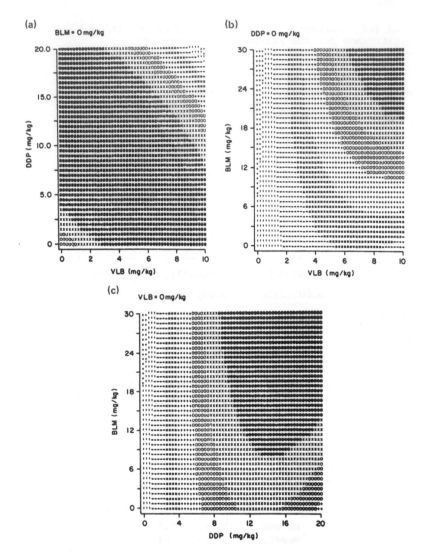

FIGURE 3.7. Plot of contours of constant relative hazard from the VLB/DDP/BLM experiment. Each graph gives the estimated relationship between two of the drugs when the third drug is given at a zero level. The range of estimated ℓn relative hazard associated with each symbol for each of the three panels as shown on page 75.

REFERENCES

1. Breslow, N. (1974). Covariance analysis of censored survival data. *Biometrics*, *30*, 89-99.

2. Breslow, N. (1975). Analysis of survival data under the proportional hazards model. *Int. Stat. Rev.*, *43*, 45-58.

3. Cox, D. R. (1972). Regression models and life tables. *J. Roy. Stat. Soc. B*, *34*, 187-220.

4. Cox, D. R. (1975). Partial likelihood. *Biometrika*, *62*, 269-276.

5. Cox, D. R., and Snell, E. (1968). A general definition of residuals. *J. Roy. Stat. Soc. B*, *30*, 248-275.

6. Efron, B. (1976). The efficiency of Cox's likelihood function for censored data. *J. Amer. Stat. Assoc.*, *72*, 557-565.

7. Feigl, P., and Zelen, M. (1965). Estimation of experimental survival probabilities with concomitant information. *Biometrics*, *21*, 826-838.

8. Glasser, M. (1967). Exponential survival with covariance. *J. Amer. Stat. Assoc.*, *62*, 561-568.

9. Kalbfleisch, J. O., and Prentice, R. L. (1972). In Discussion of regression models and life tables. *J. Roy. Stat. Soc. B*, *34*, 187-220.

10. Kalbfleisch, J. O., and Prentice, R. L. (1973). Marginal likelihood based on Cox's regression and life model. *Biometrika*, *60*, 267-278.

11. Kaplan, E. L., and Meier, P. (1958). Nonparametric estimations from incomplete observations. *J. Amer. Stat. Assoc.*, *53*, 457-481.

12. Kay, R. (1977). Proportional hazard regression models and the analysis of censored survival data. *App. Stat.*, *26*, 227-257.

13. Myers, R., Hankey, B., and Mantel, N. (1973). A logistic-exponential model for use with response time data involving regressor variables. *Biometrics*, *29*, 257-269.

14. Nelder, J. A., and Mead, R. (1965). A simplex method for function minimization. *Comp. J.*, *7*, 308-313.

15. Peace, K. E., and Flora, R. E. (1978). Size and power assessments of tests of hypothesis on survival parameters. *J. Amer. Stat. Assoc.*, *73*, 129-132.

16. Peto, R. (1972). In Discussion of regression models and
     life tables. *J. Roy. Stat. Soc. B*, *34*, 187–220.

17. Zippin, C., and Armitage, P. (1966). Use of concomitant
     variables and incomplete survival information in the
     estimation of an exponential survival parameter. *Bio-metrics*, *22*, 665–672.

4

Nonproportional Hazards

4.1 INTRODUCTION

In the previous chapter hazard-based models which assumed proportionality were examined. Substantive biologic considerations
require that this assumption be examined. In chemotherapeutic
applications it seems likely that hazard functions may not be
proportional through time. Upon treatment in the typical animal experiment, mice receiving a moderately effective therapy
should have risk, relative to the controls, which is lower at
all points later in time. On the other hand, a very effective
treatment may actually cause risk which exceeds that associated
with the control animals at early time points and which would
necessarily fall rapidly, eventually being lower than the less
effective treatment. Clinically, lethal doses of methotrexate
are administered to the patient in the surgical adjuvant treatment of osteosarcoma. Citrovorum factor rescue follows shortly
to counter the toxic effects to the host but not to the tumor.
Thus the relative hazard rises sharply, then falls. The proportional hazard model as introduced in the previous chapter
cannot be used to model such data. Thus, changes must be made
which permit the modeling of data for which the hazard functions
are nonproportional.

The changes considered here will permit the relative hazard function to be time varying, a function of treatment and time rather than treatment alone. Hence

$$\lambda(t) = \lambda_0(t) \ \exp[g(\underline{x}, \ t)]$$

For the following figure, three situations involving two treatments X_1 and X_2 and the control group X_c are considered. In Fig. 4.1A, $\exp[g(x, \ t)]$, the relative hazard function, is plotted under the proportional model. The relative hazard functions are constant in time and, as plotted, treatment X_1 is superior to both X_2 and X_c. When dealing with curable cancer it is unlikely that proportionality holds for very large t. Long-term survivors of the cancer and treatment most likely have hazard functions that are quite similar, irrespective of treatment.

Figure 4.1B describes one type of time-varying relative hazard function. Here the treatment is seen to be initially effective, while relative efficacy decreases with time. Providing that there is a treatment x_s such that

$$\exp[g(x_s, \ t)] \ \leq \ \exp[g(x_i, \ t)]$$

for every x_i and t, then location of an optimal treatment requires locating x_s. From Fig. 4.1B X_1 is clearly the best treatment considered.

A situation with more complicated relationships among the relative hazards is illustrated in Fig. 4.1C. Treatment X_1, which is actually worse than the control treatment at early time points, is superior to both the control treatment and treatment X_2 later on. The implication of crossing relative hazard functions in single-drug therapy is that no particular dose is optimal, in the sense that it maximizes the probability of survival, for every time point. Similarly, in multidrug therapies, there may be no optimal combination for all time

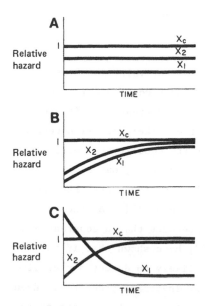

FIGURE 4.1. (A) Proportional hazards model; (B) nonproportional hazards model; (C) nonproportional hazards model crossing relative hazard functions.

points, due to the nonproportionality of the hazard functions through time. That the optimal treatment may be a function of the time interval selected may not be clinically well recognized. The crossing of relative hazard functions will lead to different treatment strategies. Decisions about whether to use treatments which are desirable for short-term effects will have to be balanced against the usefulness of therapy which increases the chance for long-term cures at the expense of fewer short-term successes.

4.2 THE TWO-TREATMENT TRIAL

Although this discussion deals primarily with the problems associated with combination chemotherapy, for simplicity, first consider a clinical trial with two treatment arms. Here the proportional hazard model is specified as

$$\lambda(t) = \lambda_0(t) \exp(x_1 \beta_1)$$

where x_1 is a dummy variable taking on the values of 0 or 1, dependent on whether the individual under consideration is a control or a treated subject. A test for treatment difference follows the maximization of the partial likelihood with respect to the parameter β_1 and testing for its equality to zero. In the absence of tied failure times, Breslow [1] has shown that this test is asymptotically equivalent to the Mantel-Haenszel or to the logrank test developed by Mantel [2]. As the model is a proportional hazards one, it presumes that a constant hazard ratio exists. Peto and Peto [3] have shown that if the model is correct, the test is more likely to detect a real difference than any other unbiased rank-invariant procedure. Even if the relative hazard function is not constant, the procedure can be used; but if the relative hazard functions intersect, either treatment may be found to be superior or no treatment difference may be determined. Thus interpretation of the test results is difficult if the relative hazard function is time varying.

As already noted, the consideration of the validity of the proportionality assumption is important. A comparison between a nonsurgical and surgical treatment is a situation in which nonproportional hazards are likely. Excess mortality associated with the surgical procedure and its complications is often observed. If this treatment arm is to be competitive, then its hazard rate must fall below that of the treatment to which it is being compared as time continues. Thus the hazard functions cross and are not proportional.

The resulting survival times of a clinical trial sponsored by the Gastro-Intestinal Tumor Study Group, an earlier analysis of which is reported on by Stablein, Carter, and Novak [4], are

TABLE 4.1. *Survival Times (Days) for Gastric Cancer Patients*

Chemotherapy		Chemotherapy and Radiation	
17	307	1	535
42	315	63	562
44	401	105	569
48	445	125	675
60	464	182	676
72	484	216	748
74	528	250	778
95	542	262	786
103	567	$301(2)^a$	797
108	577	342	955
122	580	354	968
144	795	356	977
167	855	358	1245
170	1174^+	380	1271
183	1214^+	383(2)	1420
185	1232^+	388	1460^+
193	1366	394	1516^+
195	1455^+	408	1551
197	1585^+	460	1690^+
208	1622^+	489	1694
234	1626^+	499	
235	1736^+	523	
254		524	

[a] The number in parentheses indicates the number of deaths on that day.

[+] Censored observation.

listed in Table 4.1. This study compared chemotherapy alone versus a combination of chemotherapy and radiation in the treatment of locally advanced nonresectable gastric carcinoma. In

Fig. 4.2 the product-limit estimates of the resulting survival curves are plotted.   Notice that although there is substantial separation between the estimated survival distributions at 8 to 10 months, by the twenty-sixth month the plotted curves intersect.   Although this may be the result of variability in the data, such an occurrence is not consistent with a proportional hazard model, for an implication of proportionality is that the survival distributions are powers of each other. Specifically, from Eq. (3.5)

$$S(t) = (S_0(t))^{exp(\underline{x}'\underline{\beta})}$$

and for example, when $S_0(t) = 0.7$ if $exp(\underline{x}'\beta) = 2$, then $S(t) = 0.49$ and when $S_0(t) = 0.25$, $S(t) = 0.0625$.   Notice in the above expression that the exponent of $S_0(t)$ is equal to the ratio of the hazard functions associated with the two groups.   Under the assumption of a proportional hazard model, this term must be constant over time.   From Fig. 4.2, when t equals 6 months, the

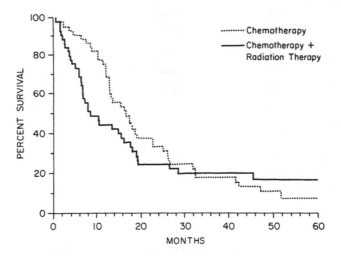

FIGURE 4.2.   *Product-limit estimates of the survival curves for the gastric carcinoma study.*

value of S(t) for the chemotherapy arm $S_1(t) = 0.911$ while the value for the combination arm $S_0(t) = 0.688$, resulting in the estimated exponent being equal to 4.012. For a larger t, in the neighborhood of 24 months, the estimated exponent is nearly 1. Thus, the widely divergent exponents make the validity of the proportional hazard assumption questionable.

Examining the results of the proportional hazard test, β_1 is estimated to be -0.141495, and the test based on asymptotic normal theory yields a p value of 0.52. Therefore, no difference between the treatment arms can be claimed. Figure 4.3 is a plot of the fitted survival distributions under the proportional hazards model. Notice that the curves are powers of each other as required by the model but that the early treatment advantage of chemotherapy alone, which can be observed in Fig. 4.2, is not at all evident in this plot. In fact, due to the evidence already gathered which indicates that the relative hazard function is not constant in time, the conclusion of no difference is suspect.

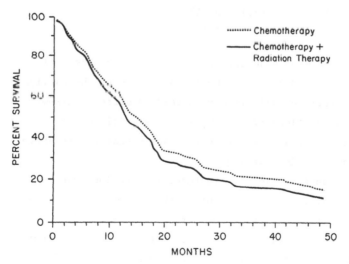

FIGURE 4.3. *Proportional hazard estimates of the survival curves for the gastric carcinoma study.*

Now consider a relative hazard function which is time varying. Let

$$\lambda(t) = \lambda_0(t) \; \exp(\beta_1 x_1 + \gamma_1 x_1 t^*)$$

where t^* is t measured in days divided by 30. Thus a time by treatment interaction has been introduced into the model. Significance testing of the hypothesis that $\gamma_1 = 0$ will yield an indication of the reasonableness of the proportionality assumption.

Estimation of the parameters will require, as before, the maximization of the partial likelihood function

$$L = \prod_{j=1}^{k} \frac{\Pi_{i=1}^{m_j} \exp(\beta_1 x_i + \gamma_1 x_i t_j^*)}{\Sigma_{s \in R(t_j)} \exp(\beta_1 x_1 + \gamma_1 x_s t_j^*)^{m_j}} \tag{4.1}$$

with respect to β_1 and γ_1.

The estimates and their estimated asymptotic standard errors obtained when analyzing this trial are determined to be

$$\hat{\beta}_1 = -1.2711 \qquad \hat{SE}(\hat{\beta}_1) = 0.419$$
$$\hat{\gamma}_1 = 0.0794 \qquad \hat{SE}(\hat{\gamma}_1) = 0.026$$

The test for treatment equality $H_0: (\beta_1, \gamma_1) = \underline{0}$ yields a likelihood ratio $\chi_2^2 = 13.48$, $p = 0.0012$. As a result, the survival curves by the refined analysis can be said to differ. Likewise, the test for proportionality $H_0: \gamma_1 = 0$ is significant ($p < 0.001$), and there is a very strong indication that the relative hazard function is time varying.

The importance of time by treatment interactions can be viewed in Fig. 4.4. This is a plot of the estimated log relative hazard function for the chemotherapy arm versus time enclosed by its associated 95% confidence interval. Recall that the log relative hazard for the combined modality equals 0 by

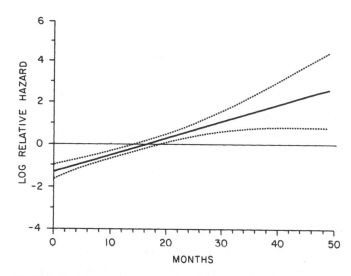

FIGURE 4.4. *Estimated relative hazard function for the chemo-therapy arm in the gastric carcinoma study and associated 95% confidence limits.*

definition. If the plotted curve in Fig. 4.4 equals 0 for every t, then $\lambda(t) - \lambda_0(t)$ and the two treatment groups have identical survival distributions. Marked differences in the treatment effects as evidenced in this figure are observed. Note that at the start the relative hazard for the chemotherapy arm is sig-nificantly lower than that for the group that received the com-bination. By 15 months the relative hazard functions cross and as time increases, the chemotherapy arm has associated with it a significantly higher hazard than that of the combined modality arm. As time progresses there is increasing variability in the estimated relative hazard. The magnitude of the estimated func-tion at various time points is rather impressive, the chemother-apy arm being nearly 3.5 times better than the combination at the beginning of the trial. Unfortunately, the treatment advan-tage reverses and by the study's end the relative risk of being on the drug-only arm is nearly 10; i.e., at the study's end

those who received chemotherapy alone are almost 10 times more
likely to fail at a given instant in time than those who received the combination. This is evidence of the magnitude of
the nonproportionality of the hazard functions. Note further
that the relative hazard from the proportional model yields the
discrepant result of an estimated relative instantaneous risk
for the combination versus chemotherapy of exp(0.1415) = 1.15
at all time points.

Plotting the estimated survival distributions, one obtains
Fig. 4.5. In contrast to Fig. 4.3, note the marked similarity
the modeled distributions have to those estimated separately
for the two treatment groups in Fig. 4.2. The nonproportional
model clearly represents the data more faithfully. The results
of this analysis then clearly indicate that these survival distributions differ. In fact, they differ in that the combined
modality arm has a high early mortality. As time goes on its
associated hazard function becomes less than that of the

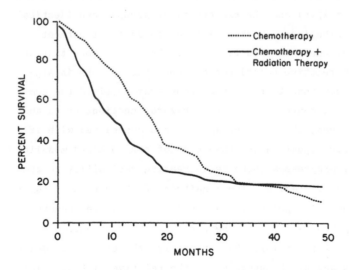

FIGURE 4.5. *Nonproportional hazard estimates of the survival*
curves for the gastric carcinoma study.

chemotherapy group, and while the fact that the estimated survival curves cross late in the course of the study is encourag-
ing, it is not conclusive evidence of cumulative combination
superiority.

4.3 NONPROPORTIONALITY IN COMBINATION EXPERIMENTS

From the clinical trial just examined, it is clear that different treatments do not always yield survival distributions with
proportional hazards. The proportionality assumption should
also be assessed with regard to the many survival curves resulting from a combination experiment. For two drugs x_1 and x_2 a
reasonable relationship might be

$$g(x, \ t) = \underline{x}'\underline{\beta} + \gamma_1 x_1 t + \gamma_2 x_2 t + \gamma_{11} x_1 t^2 + \gamma_{22} x_2 t^2$$

where $\underline{x}'\underline{\beta}$ is a full quadratic in x_1 and x_2. This model for the
log relative hazard has interaction of treatment with both time
and time squared. Although the interaction with time alone may
be sufficient (as in the previous example), the above model provides for additional flexibility among the hazard functions.
Additionally, it is the simplest polynomial relationship that
permits curvature through time of the relative hazard functions.
Parameter estimation can proceed by modifying the likelihood
function of Eq. (4.1) to incorporate the desired relative hazard
function. Due to the time-varying nature of the relative hazard,
contour plots of this function are not as useful as in the proportional hazard situation. A set of plots could be generated
for each instant in time. Further, the effect of the relative
hazard on the survival distribution is dependent on both the
underlying hazard and the size of the population of survivors.
Neither of these can be incorporated into the relative hazard
plots, and their usefulness in these analyses is limited.

Proceeding with the analysis requires an estimate of the underlying hazard function. Following the developments of Sect. 3.5, an estimate conditional on the parameter estimates can be obtained at the days of death as

$$\lambda_0(t_j) = \frac{m_j}{\int_{t_{j-1}}^{t_j} \Sigma_{i \in R(t_j)} \exp(\underline{x}_i'\hat{\underline{\beta}} + \hat{\gamma}_1 x_1 u + \hat{\gamma}_2 x_2 u + \hat{\gamma}_{11} x_1 u^2 + \hat{\gamma}_{22} x_2 u^2) \, du}$$

The function has constant value in the interval (t_{j-1}, t_j). Notice that the hazard function for all other treatment combinations, since each is a multiple of $\lambda_0(t)$, will be continuous and time varying between days of death with point discontinuities at times of death.

Further information can be extracted from the experiment by examining the response surface delineated by the parameter estimates. For k drugs, the nonproportional model describes a surface in k + 2 dimensions. An optimal dose can be defined as that which maximizes the estimated probability of survival to time t,

$$\max_{\underline{x}} \exp\left\{-\int_0^t \hat{\lambda}_0(u) \, \exp[\hat{g}(x, u)] \, du\right\}$$

$$= \min_{\underline{x}} \int_0^t \hat{\lambda}_0(u) \, \exp[\hat{g}(\underline{x}, u)] \, du \tag{4.2}$$

so that the optimal dose is a function of the time interval selected. The solution of the above may require numerical integration.

Equation (4.2) provides some insight into the models discussed in previous chapters. A major problem with the application of the logistic analysis is the need to define failures and successes. The result of changing definitions would be changes in the dose estimated to be the optimum.

The proportional hazard model avoids this difficulty and estimates the unique optimal treatment combination. If in fact there is nonproportionality, there may not exist a single optimum, but under Eq. (4.2) the optimal combination is a function of the desired interval. From this view, the unique optimum does not exist, but rather the optimum varies with different treatment strategies. Thus, through refinement of the proportional hazard model, a return to a time-dependent definition of success as espoused in the logistic model is achieved. Clearly, clinical decision-making with well-understood treatment may involve the selection of a treatment strategy. Unfortunately, we can not endorse a priori a single method of determining an optimal strategy, since an optimal strategy is a value-dependent entity. Estimating the strategy which maximizes mean survival time may be statistically simple, but this simplicity may overshadow the fact that implicit value statements are incorporated in its development. Ethical arguments can be made relating its advantages in clinical situations to those of maximizing long-term survivors, median survival time, or short-term benefits. The results of such discussions will often be disease- and treatment-dependent, and further exploration of such issues will not be pursued here.

The assessment of model fit involves the comparison of the empirical survival distributions with the fitted distributions. Notice that the rank-correlation coefficients appropriate for the proportional model are no longer applicable measures of fit. This is due to the changing relationships among the relative hazard functions, which no longer imply a constant ordering of the median survival times. Standard goodness of fit criteria for relating the two distributions may not be applicable, due to the small sample sizes at each treatment point, but visual inspection for model deficiencies is possible. Residual analysis can proceed as before, with the more general definition of the residuals being

$$\varepsilon_i = \int_0^{t_i} \exp[g(\underline{x}_i, u)] \lambda_0(u) \, du$$

4.4 ANALYSIS OF EXPERIMENTAL DATA

For clarity we will begin with the analysis of a two-drug experiment. As in the typical chemotherapy animal survival study,
this experiment began with the injection of malignant tumor
cells into a batch of mice. Two hundred sixteen B6D2F$_1$ female
mice were injected intraperitoneally with 10^5 L1210 leukemia
cells. The design used eight animals per group in a 5^2 factorial arrangement augmented with two high-dose single-drug treatments. Treatment consisted of administration of two drugs,
($\pm$)-1,2-bis(3,5-dioxopiperazin-1-yl)propane (ICRF-159) and
hexamethylmelamine (HXM), four times daily on days 7, 11, and
15 after tumor inoculation. Deaths were recorded daily and the
experiment was terminated on day 50. The treatment groups and
resulting survival times are included in Table 4.2.

*TABLE 4.2. Treatment and Survival Data and Fitted Quartiles
from the Nonproportional Model for the ICRF-159/HXM Experiment*

Treatment (mg/kg)			Fitted quartiles from nonproportional model		
ICRF-159	HXM	Survival times (days)	q.25	q.50	q.75
0.00	0.00	9,10(2),11(5)[a]	10.0	10.3	10.8
50.00	0.00	11,12(2),13(2),15,16,22	10.7	11.9	13.3
75.00	0.00	12(2),13(2),14,21,23(2)	11.4	13.0	18.1
112.50	0.00	13(3),14(2),22(2),24	12.7	19.5	24.0
169.00	0.00	11,12,13,23,24,27,30,33	15.6	23.8	26.5
253.00	0.00	14,23,24,25,26(2),29,37	22.4	24.5	27.4
0.00	20.00	10(4),11(4)	10.1	10.7	11.8

TABLE 4.2 continued

Treatment (mg/kg)			Fitted quartiles from nonproportional model		
ICRF-159	HXM	Survival times (days)	q.25	q.50	q.75
0.00	30.00	10(2),11(6)	10.2	11.0	12.3
0.00	45.00	11(7),50[+]	10.3	11.3	12.9
0.00	67.50	11(6),13,14	10.4	11.6	13.4
0.00	101.00	11(4),12(3),15	10.1	10.9	12.5
50.00	20.00	13(3),14,21,23,24,25	11.3	13.0	21.4
50.00	30.00	11(2),12,14(2),20,24	11.6	13.6	23.5
50.00	45.00	11,15,23,25,26,29,30,24	11.9	14.6	25.0
50.00	67.50	12,15(2),24,25(3),26	11.9	17.1	27.2
75.00	20.00	12(2),13(3),14,15,24	12.2	15.0	24.2
75.00	30.00	14,24,25,26(2),29,30,39	12.5	22.0	25.6
75.00	45.00	24(2),25,26,27,28,29,32	12.9	23.5	28.4
75.00	67.50	14(2),15,17,29(3),33	12.9	23.3	29.9
112.50	20.00	8,10,13(2),24,25,29,31	13.8	23.7	27.7
112.50	30.00	13(2),24(2),25,26,36(2)	14.5	24.6	29.3
112.50	45.00	11,16,26(2),27(2),33,35	16.5	25.8	31.4
112.50	67.50	14(2),30(2),32,33,38,42	15.5	26.7	32.1
169.00	20.00	12(3),14,15,25,28	22.9	25.7	30.3
169.00	30.00	13,14,24(2),26,29,31,50[+]	23.3	26.8	31.8
169.00	45.00	12,25,27(2),28,31,35,50[+]	23.6	20.2	32.6
169.00	67.50	11,15,16,18,31(2),32,33	23.4	28.2	32.2

[a]The number in parentheses indicates the number of deaths on that day.

[+]Censored observation.

Source: Reproduced from: Stablein, D. M., Carter, W. H., Jr., and Wampler, G. L. (1980). Survival analysis of drug combinations using a hazards model with time-dependent covariates. *Biometrics*, *36*, 537–546. With permission of The Biometric Society.

TABLE 4.3. *Parameter Estimates, Standard Errors, and Significance for the Proportional and Nonproportional Hazard Models*

	Proportional hazard model				Nonproportional hazard model		
Parameter	Estimate	Standard error	Significance	Parameter	Estimate	Standard error	Significance
β_1 (ICRF-159)	-0.025808	0.004590	p < 0.0001	β_1	-0.031260	0.005575	p < 0.0001
β_2 (HXM)	-0.049260	0.012610	p < 0.0001	β_2	-0.022128	0.013172	p = 0.0930
β_{11}	0.000062	0.000016	p < 0.0010	β_{11}	0.000106	0.000071	p = 0.1355
β_{22}	0.000378	0.000101	p < 0.0002	β_{22}	0.000057	0.000020	p = 0.0044
β_{12}	0.000093	0.000049	p < 0.06	β_{12}	0.000277	0.000105	p = 0.0084
				γ_{11}	0.000180	0.000752	p = 0.8109
				γ_{12}	-0.004561	0.001938	p = 0.0186
				γ_{21}	0.000012	0.000024	p = 0.6170
				γ_{22}	0.000158	0.000065	p = 0.0151

Source: Reproduced from Stablein, D. M., Carter, W. H., Jr., and Wampler, G. L. (1980). Survival analysis of drug combinations using a hazards model with time-dependent covariates. *Biometrics, 36,* 537–546. With permission of The Biometric Society.

The variables x_1 and x_2 were set equal to the doses of
ICRF-159 and HXM in mg/kg, respectively, while time was scaled
in days such that $t = 0$ corresponded to day 7, the day of ini-
tiation of therapy. Table 4.3 includes the parameter estimates
and their estimated standard errors under both the proportional
and the nonproportional models. The likelihood-ratio criterion
for inclusion of the time parameters γ, a test of proportionality, yields a highly significant $\chi_4^2 = 32.52$, $p < 0.0001$.

A survival curve was estimated for each treatment using
$\hat{\lambda}(t)$ and the relationship between survival distributions and
hazard functions. Since the group sizes are too small to con-
fidently apply a χ^2 test of fit, a one-sample Kolmogorov-Smirnov
test was applied to compare each empirical distribution to its
estimated survival distribution. This was done despite the in-
ability of this test to compensate for the fitted parameters.
None of the 27 distributions result in the rejection of the
hypothesis of equality at the 0.05 level. Likewise, inspection
of the fitted distribution quartiles listed in Table 4.2 provide no indications of systematic departures from the model.
Thus there is no evidence that the fit is inadequate, and further exploration of the response surface seems reasonable.

Figure 4.6, a contour plot, is a projection of the rela-
tive hazard function $\exp(\underline{x}'\hat{\underline{\beta}})$, estimated under the proportional
model, onto the ICRF-159, HXM plane. The estimated optimum
doses are: ICRF-159 = 175.8 mg/kg and HXM = 43.5 mg/kg. The
corresponding height of the surface is .035, while the estimated median survival time is 27 days.

The nonproportional model is used to estimate the optimal
treatment combinations for various time intervals which are
plotted in Fig. 4.7. Contrary to what may be expected, the
trace of the optima through time indicates that the chance for
long-term survival improves by increasing the dosage of HXM,
an inactive drug when given alone, and by actually decreasing
the dosage of ICRF-159. To verify this result, a repeat exper-

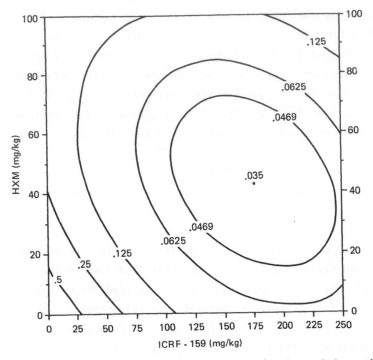

FIGURE 4.6. *Contours of constant relative hazard from the ICRF-159/HXM treatment of advanced L1210 leukemia. (Reproduced from: Stablein, D. M., Carter, W. H., Jr., and Wampler, G. L. (1980). Survival analysis of drug combinations using a hazards model with time-dependent covariates. Biometrics 36, 537-546. With permission of The Biometric Society.)*

iment was run with doses of ICRF-159 ranging up to 250 mg/kg, the higher doses to ensure that the optimal treatments were within the experimental region. Tests based on the asymptotic normality of γ_{11} and γ_{21} yielded significance at the 0.01 level, and a similar tracing of the optima through time resulted.

The plots of the survival distributions for several treatment combinations are included in Fig. 4.8. Notice that despite the statistical importance of γ, the treatment by time interactions, the difference in survival distributions which maximize 13-day and 29-day survival are small until day 22. Likewise, the survival curve for the optima from the proportional analy-

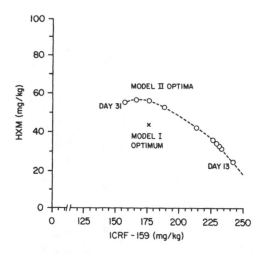

FIGURE 4.7. *Trace of optimal treatment combinations for various time intervals from the nonproportional hazards analysis of the ICRF-159/HXM experiment. Model I is a proportional hazards model and Model II is a nonproportional hazards model. (Reproduced from: Stablein, D. M., Carter, W. H., Jr., and Wampler, G. L. Survival analysis of drug combinations using a hazards model with time-dependent covariates. Biometrics, 36, 537-546. With permission of The Biometric Society.)*

sis is similar to both.

While the statistical significance of γ verifies the nonproportionality of the hazard functions, the implications for treatment of the animal tumor are not necessarily substantially different from the results obtained with the proportional hazard model. Comparison of Figs. 4.6 and 4.7 point to both procedures' ability to estimate similar successful treatment regions. However, the nonproportional model provides additional information on the combined action of the drugs used. These drug relationships estimated from an in vivo mammalian tumor system may well be more useful in extrapolation to human disease than the actual optimum doses.

Consider now a three-drug regimen. The drugs cyclophosphamide (Cytoxan; CTX), mitomycin-C (MIT), and mechlorethamine (nitrogen mustard; HN2) were tested for their antineoplastic

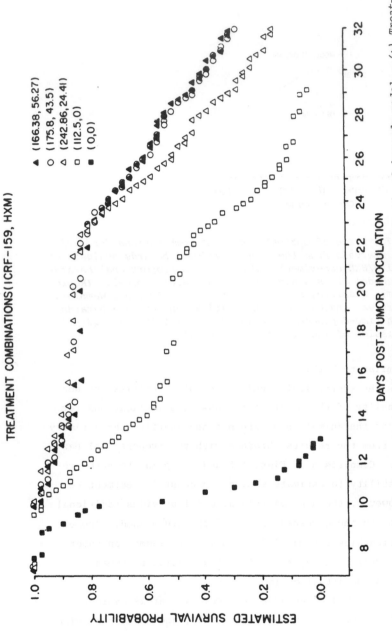

FIGURE 4.8. Survival distributions estimated from the nonproportional hazards model. (▲) Treatment associated with the 29-day optimum; (△) treatment associated with the 13-day optimum; (○) treatment associated with the proportional hazards optimum. (Reproduced from: Stablein, D. M., Carter, W. H., Jr., and Wampler, G. L. (1980). Survival analysis of drug combinations using a hazards model with time-dependent covariates. Biometrics, 36, 537–546. (With permission of The Biometrics Society.)

effects in combination against P388 murine leukemia. B6D2F$_1$
mice with an average weight of 22.2 g were used. A single injection of drugs was administered on day 0 when the day of tumor
inoculation with 10^6 cells i.p. occurred seven days previously.
The treatment combination and survival times are given in Table
4.4. In the analysis, drug dosages were scaled such that

$$x_1 = \frac{\text{dose CTX, mg/kg}}{400}$$

$$x_2 = \frac{\text{dose MIT, mg/kg}}{10}$$

$$x_3 = \frac{\text{dose HN2, mg/kg}}{4}$$

Applying the proportional hazard analysis using a full quadratic model, one obtains the parameter estimates given in Table
4.5. Notice that significant beneficial and harmful effects
are associated with each drug. Table 4.6 is included to demonstrate model fit, while contour plots of the relative hazard
function are included in Fig. 4.9. The optimum dose is estimated to be CTX 200 mg/kg, MIT 0.0 mg/kg, and HN2 2.2 mg/kg.

A nonproportional model with six additional parameters
for the interaction of dose with t and t^2 is now presented.
The maximum-likelihood estimates and their standard deviations
are listed in Table 4.7. Notice that asymptotic normality
tests for five of the six time-related parameters are significant at the 0.01 level of significance. The likelihood-ratio
test for $\underline{\gamma} = \underline{0}$ yields a $\chi_6^2 = 41.81$ (p < 0.001).

Turning to an appraisal of the goodness of fit of the proportional model, inspection shows that the cumulative hazard
residual plot in Fig. 4.10 is not indicative of departure from
an underlying unit exponential error distribution. A one-sample
Kolmogorov-Smirnov test rejects the fit for treatment 24 at the
0.05 level. Six of eight animals had died by day 12 (one was
censored and the other died on day 25) but the estimate of the

TABLE 4.4.   Treatment and Survival Data from
CTX/MIT/HN2 Experiment

Treatment (mg/kg)			
CTX	MIT	HN2	Survival time (days)
0.00	0.00	0.00	$8(3)^a,9(5)$
87.00	0.00	0.00	9,11(2),12(3),24,31
218.00	0.00	0.00	11,31(3),32,34(2),37
392.00	0.00	0.00	8(5),11,12(2)
0.00	2.60	0.00	8(2),9,11,12,16
0.00	6.50	0.00	8,10,11,12(3),17,19
0.00	11.70	0.00	11,12(3),13,15
0.00	0.00	0.87	10,11(5),12,15
0.00	0.00	2.18	11(4),12(2),13(2)
0.00	0.00	3.92	11(2),13,15(4),17
34.80	1.04	0.35	9(2),11(3),12(2),20
218.00	1.04	0.35	10,30,42,51,56,60$^+$(3)
34.80	6.50	0.35	8,11(2),12,17,23,24,34
34.80	1.04	2.18	9,11(2),12(2),21,24,25
218.00	6.50	0.35	10,13,14,31,32,60$^+$(3)
218.00	1.04	2.18	11,15,34,60$^+$(5)
34.80	6.50	2.18	11,12(6),17
218.00	6.50	2.18	13(4),15(4)
392.00	2.60	0.87	7,8(5),10,12
17.40	2.60	0.87	11,12(2),13,20(2),25,42
87.00	11.70	0.87	9(2),11,12(2),13(2),15
87.00	0.52	0.87	9,26,27(2),28,31,32,34
87.00	2.60	3.92	12,13(3),15(3),29
87.00	2.60	0.17	8,11(2),12(3),25,60$^+$
87.00	2.60	0.87	11(2),12,26,29,30,42,60$^+$

^{a}The number in parentheses indicates the number
of deaths on that day.
$^+$Censored observation.

TABLE 4.5. *Parameter Estimates, Standard Errors, and
Significance for the CTX/MIT/HN2 P388 Experiment*

Parameter	Maximum-likelihood estimate	Standard error	Significance
β_1 (CTX)	-13.45	1.36	$p < 0.001$
β_2 (MIT)	-4.77	0.93	$p < 0.001$
β_3 (HN2)	-5.39	1.15	$p < 0.001$
β_{11}	13.01	1.29	$p < 0.001$
β_{22}	2.81	0.72	$p < 0.001$
β_{33}	3.45	1.03	$p < 0.001$
β_{12}	4.54	1.26	$p < 0.001$
β_{13}	2.92	1.52	$p < 0.06$
β_{23}	7.67	1.33	$p < 0.001$

survival distribution on day 12 is 0.707. Thus, this particular
fitted survival distribution fails to fall rapidly enough in
the early days. The fit for all remaining 24 treatment groups
is adequate at the 0.10 level by this test.

Although the test for proportionality has already indicated the necessity of the additional parameters, it may be interesting to compare the two models' fit in this data set. One
such comparison would be to calculate the number of treatments
for which the nonproportional model gives a better fit, i.e.,

$$Y = \sum_{treatments} y_i$$

where

$$y_i = 1 \quad \text{if } D_{max\ i}\ \text{nonprop} < D_{max\ i}\ \text{prop}$$
$$\quad = 0 \quad \text{otherwise}$$

and

TABLE 4.6. *Ranking of Median Survival Times and
Estimated Hazards for Treatment Groups in CTX/MIT/HN2
Experiment*

Treatment group[a]	Rank of median survival time	Rank of estimated hazard
1	3.0	2
2	11.0	16
3	22.5	21
4	1.5	3
5	4.0	5
6	11.0	13
7	11.0	8
8	5.5	4
9	7.0	12
10	18.0	10
11	5.5	11
12	24.0	24
13	17.0	17
14	11.0	18
15	22.5	22
16	25.0	25
17	11.0	7
18	15.5	9
19	1.5	1
20	19.0	14
21	11.0	6
22	20.5	20
23	15.5	15
24	11.0	19
25	20.5	23

[a]For treatments see Table 4.4.

Spearman's $\hat{\rho}$ = 0.8465 (p < 0.001).

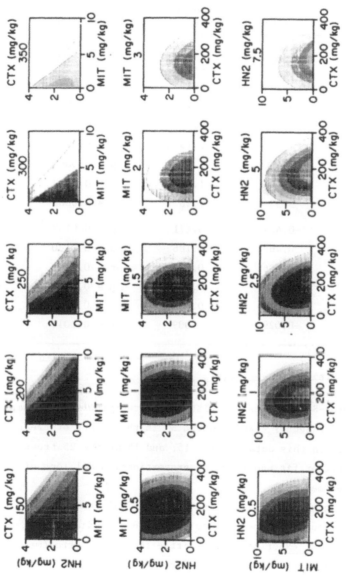

FIGURE 4.9. Contour plots of the relative hazard function from the CTX/MIT/HN2 experiment. (The darker the shading, the lower the value of the relative hazard.) (From Carter, W. H., Jr., Stablein, D. M., and Wampler, G. L. (1979). An improved method for analyzing survival data from combination chemotherapy experiments, Cancer Res., 39, 3446-3453.)

TABLE 4.7. Nonproportional Hazard Model Parameter Estimates and Estimated Standard Errors for CTX/MIT/HN2 Treatment of Advanced P388 Leukemia Experiment

Parameter	Estimate	Standard error	Significance
β_1 (CTX)	-9.87	1.62	$p < 0.0001$
β_2 (MIT)	-5.57	1.13	$p < 0.0001$
β_3 (HN2)	-7.33	1.31	$p < 0.0001$
β_{11}	10.56	1.42	$p < 0.0001$
β_{22}	2.26	0.76	$p = 0.0030$
β_{33}	2.30	1.15	$p = 0.0455$
β_{12}	5.47	1.45	$p = 0.0002$
β_{13}	2.49	1.79	$p = 0.1642$
β_{23}	5.53	1.46	$p = 0.0002$
γ_{11}	-0.424	0.171	$p = 0.0132$
γ_{12}	0.462	0.186	$p = 0.0130$
γ_{13}	0.806	0.223	$p = 0.0003$
γ_{21}	0.011	0.006	$p = 0.0668$
γ_{22}	-0.020	0.007	$p = 0.0043$
γ_{23}	-0.029	0.009	$p = 0.0013$

$$D_{max} = S(t)_{empirical} - S(t)_{fitted}$$

the Kolmogorov-Smirnov test statistic. If the fit is the same, then we would expect $Y = NG/2$, where NG is the number of treatment groups. In this data set $Y = 15$, and 15 of the 25 treatments have better fit under the nonproportional model (one of which is treatment 24).

A listing of the optimum doses for survival from day 7 to day i for various i is included in Table 4.8. Notice, in contrast to the last experiment, how little the optimal treatments change with time as well as how similar they are to the optimum from the proportional analysis. Again a zero dose of MIT seems

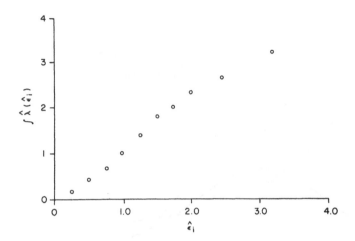

FIGURE 4.10. *Estimated cumulative hazard function for the nonproportional hazards model analysis of the CTX/MIT/HN2 experiment.*

appropriate. In Fig. 4.11, the relative hazard function is plotted for several treatments to investigate the relative value of MIT and HN2. It is interesting to speculate on the causes of the observed relationships. One possibility is that in combination with CTX a dose of HN2 has more substantial antitumor effect in the early time periods than does MIT. Giving 2 units of MIT along with the optimal combination has little effect in the first few days but increases the relative hazard in later days. Not too surprisingly, 30-day survivors

TABLE 4.8. *Estimated Optimal Treatments for Various Time Intervals in the P388 Experiment*

Drug	Day 7 to 13	Day 7 to 17	Day 7 to 21	Day 7 to 25
CTX	199.4	200.2	198.9	218.0
MIT	0.0	0.0	0.0	0.0
HN2	2.8	2.4	2.2	2.1

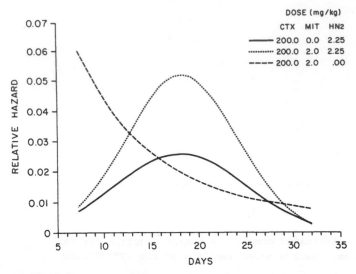

FIGURE 4.11. *Estimated relative hazard functions for three treatment combinations from the nonproportional hazards analysis of the CTX/MIT/HN2 experiment.*

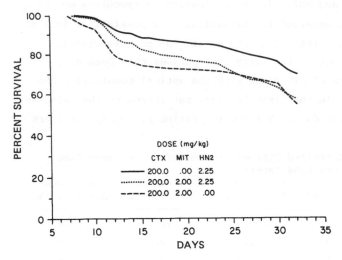

FIGURE 4.12. *Estimated survival distributions for three treatment combinations from the nonproportional hazards analysis of the CTX/MIT/HN2 experiment.*

have comparable hazards no matter what the treatment, since these animals are all effectively treatment successes. Plots of the survival distributions for these same treatments are included in Fig. 4.12. The crossing of survival distributions observed in the figure is possible if the proportionality assumption is removed. It is estimated that the two treatments containing MIT, despite the substantial differences in their relative hazard functions, have a nearly identical percentage of survival at 32 days past tumor inoculation.

REFERENCES

1. Breslow, N. (1975). Analysis of survival data under the proportional hazards model. *Int. Stat. Rev.*, *43*, 45-58.

2. Mantel, N. (1966). Evaluation of survival data and two new rank order statistics arising in its consideration. *Cancer Chemother. Rep.*, *50*, 163-170.

3. Peto, R., and Peto, J. (1972). Asymptotically efficient rank invariant test procedures (with discussion). *J. Roy. Stat. Soc. A*, *135*, 185-206.

4. Stablein, D. M., Carter, W. H., and Novak, J. W. (1981). Analysis of survival data with nonproportional hazard functions. *Cont. Clin. Trials*, *2*, 149-159.

5

Experimental Design

5.1 INTRODUCTION

The rationale behind the design of animal experiments to evaluate the effectiveness of drug combinations appears to be derived from that developed by Goldin et al. [3] for the evaluation of single drugs. Basically, the drug is administered on
a given schedule to groups of 5 to 10 diseased animals at a
number of different dosage levels, and the survival time of
each animal is recorded. The purpose of these experiments is
to demonstrate activity against a particular tumor and to determine the optimum dose for the given schedule of administration. In these experiments the determination of the optimal
treatment level is made by a visual inspection of the data,
e.g., a plot of the median survival time against dosage level.
From such a plot it is possible to discern the dose response
(survival time) curve. At the ineffective low levels of treatment the median survival times do not differ greatly from that
of the untreated control animals, but as dosage levels increase
toward the optimum there is a corresponding increase in the
median survival time. Once the optimal dosage level is exceeded
a decrease in the median survival time occurs due to the toxic
effects of the drug. It should be obvious that the accurate

estimation of the optimal dosage level determined by such a procedure depends upon an experimental design which requires a large number of closely spaced treatment levels, ranging from the untreated control group to drug levels high enough to produce visible toxicity.

When two drugs are considered in combination, it is important to determine if a therapeutic synergism occurs. Under the definition of Venditti et al. [9] such a synergism is said to exist if the combination yields a treatment which is more effective than that which can be delivered by either drug alone. Once a therapeutic synergism is demonstrated it is important to determine the optimal combination. The ray design, given in Fig. 5.1A, used by Goldin and described by Mantel [5] in the study of two drugs, involved using combinations in which the

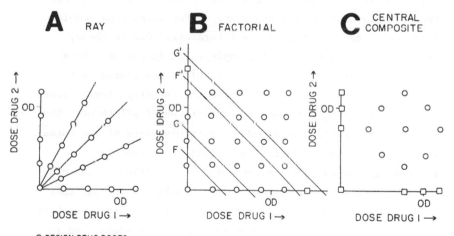

FIGURE 5.1. *Graphic representation of various experimental designs for two drugs.*

two drugs were present in a fixed ratio at several different
dosage levels. Dosage levels were fixed since at a fixed ratio
the combination can be considered as a single drug which then
permits an analysis based on the same principles as that associated with single-drug experiments. The treatment space is
effectively covered by considering various drug ratios. Other
commonly used designs in the evaluation of two-drug combinations are the 5^2, given in Fig. 5.1B, and 6^2 factorial
experiments.

For experiments dealing with three-drug combinations the
design problem is not so easily solved. In such designs the
number of treatment groups becomes large, e.g., for a 5^3 factorial experiment 125 treatment groups would be needed. With
6 animals per group such an experiment would require 750 animals. Experiments this large are generally not feasible as a
result of their expense and the strain on personnel and facil-
ities required to handle such a large number of animals. For
these and perhaps other reasons only a few three-drug combinations have been reported in the literature. One of these,
described by Goldin et al. [4] employed an ingenious scheme
for arriving at the treatment combinations considered in the
experiment. The design involved testing the drugs given alone,
in combinations of two, and in combinations of all three. The
two-drug combinations involved all possible pairs of the three
drugs, with varying ratios between pairs. In tests of the
three-drug combinations the percentage composition of the drugs
in the combined therapy varied. These authors point out that
any given design using their methodology is equivalent to choos-
ing treatment points at the vertices, along the edges, and in
the interior of an equilateral triangle. The geometry of this
figure shows that each point can be used to identify the relative proportion in which the drugs are used in the combination.

After considering different drug ratios and dosage levels, this experiment required 149 different treatment groups, including the untreated control group. Using 5 to 6 animals per group led to an experiment requiring between 750 and 900 animals. The analysis was also a visual assessment of the relationships among the median survival times for the different treatment groups. While it may be possible to extend this type of design to situations in which it is desired to study more drugs in combination, there is no motivation to do so, due to the large numbers of animals required.

Wampler, Carter, and Williams [10] have used the central composite design described by Box and Wilson [1] to evaluate drug combinations in animal experiments. Central composite designs were developed to provide enough treatment combinations to permit the estimation of the parameters in a quadratic predictive model, while using considerably fewer treatment groups than other experimental designs previously espoused. A central composite design in a k-drug combination uses $2^k + 2k + 1$ treatment combinations. If an untreated control group is used there are $2^k + 2k + 2$ treatment groups. An attractive feature associated with central composite designs derives from the use of fractional replication of the 2^k factorial component of the design when the number of drugs used becomes large. The obvious importance of the central composite design is that it makes experiments with many treatment variables possible in the laboratory and in the clinical setting. We have found it desirable to augment the design with single-drug controls as shown in Fig. 5.1C. Figures 5.1A, B, and C provide a visual comparison of the various designs that have been described for two-drug combinations. It should be noted that the design for a three-drug combination developed by Goldin et al. is a modified ray design where four doses are placed on each ray in addition to the control and where there are 3 single-drug rays, 15 two-drug rays,

and 19 three-drug rays. In addition to varying angles between
rays, their design differed from that inferred from Fig. 5.1A
in that the incremental doses on each ray are on a plane rather
than on arcs of a sphere. The many possibilities for variation
in the design of these experiments automatically lead to the
question of which design is best or, alternatively, to a consideration of the advantages and disadvantages of each type of
design.

When the form of an underlying model is assumed, design
considerations should be forthcoming from examination of the
model. For example, in a linear model of the form $\underline{y} = X\underline{\beta} + \underline{\varepsilon}$,
the parameter estimates $\hat{\underline{\beta}}$, as well as their variances, can be
analytically solved for. The parameter estimates are $\hat{\underline{\beta}} =$
$(X'X)^{-1}X'y$ and var $\hat{\underline{\beta}} = \sigma^2(X'X)^{-1}$. As it is desirable to have
little variability in the distribution of the parameter esti-
mates, design points can be selected so as to make the diagonal
elements of $(X'X)^{-1}$ small. Thus, the quality of the design, at
least as regards the variability of the parameter estimates,
can be analytically assessed.

In the proportional hazard analysis, where the response,
hazard, is not actually observed, problems with the analytic
determination of design criteria are immediately encountered.
Parameters are estimated by maximum-likelihood methods and are
solutions to Eq. (3.8). Neither the parameter estimates nor
their statistical properties can be obtained in closed form.
Thus, analytic expressions for the effect of design on the
estimates from this model are not available and Monte Carlo
simulation studies are required to provide answers to questions
concerning the proper design for survival experiments.

5.2 RESOURCE ALLOCATION

Among the design questions that need to be answered is one concerning how to best allocate available resources, e.g., in an experiment with a fixed number of experimental units is it better to heavily replicate relatively few treatment combinations or to increase the number of treatment combinations considered at the expense of the replication. Stablein [7] considered this question in a simulation study of animal experiments involving a single drug and two-drug combinations. The model assumed in this study was one of proportional hazards, i.e.,

$$\lambda(t) = \lambda_0(t) \ \exp(\underline{x}'\underline{\beta})$$

For the simulations the underlying hazard $\lambda_0(t)$ was taken to be that of the Weibull distribution, since it permits the generation of distributions with increasing, decreasing, and constant hazard functions. In the study the true response surface, and the fitted surface, was a full quadratic in the drugs administered $\underline{x}$, e.g., in the case of a single drug $\underline{x}'\underline{\beta} = \beta_1 x_1 + \beta_{11} x_1^2$.

In animal experiments the survival data are often grouped, since any subject who died after the inspection on day J is considered to have survived at least until day J + 1. In addition to grouping, data from these experiments are frequently incomplete as a result of right-single censoring. Such censoring occurs when the experiment is terminated prior to the failure of all experimental subjects.

In his study Stablein used grouped, censored data which were analyzed to determine the effect of different designs. After specifying the survival distribution, the hazard surface via the model parameters, the amounts of grouping and censoring, and the design points (i.e., treatment levels), survival data were generated using a uniform (0, 1) random number generator. Thus the ungrouped survival times were obtained from the transformation $F_i^{-1}(v)$, where $F_i = 1 - S_i$, S_i is the survival distribution associated with the ith treatment group, and v is a uniform (0, 1) random deviate. For each different set of experimental conditions, 400 different sets of experimental data were generated for the single-drug simulation while 300 different sets of data were generated for the two-drug study. This disparity was caused by the different number of observations in the experiment required to model a single-drug and a two-drug experiment. Using the methods discussed in Chap. 3, the model parameters $\underline{\beta}$, an optimal dose X_{opt}, and the response at the optimum Y_{opt} were estimated. From these the average values of $\hat{\underline{\beta}}$, $\hat{X}_{opt}$, and $\hat{Y}_{opt}$ were calculated; since their true values were known, the mean squared error (MSE), variance, and bias were determined. For this application

$$MSE = \sum_{i=1}^{N} \frac{(\hat{\theta}_i - \theta)^2}{N}$$

where

$\hat{\theta}_i$ = ith value of the estimate of parameter θ

N = number of repetitions of the simulated experiment

This statistic was chosen because it is a measure of the closeness of the estimate to the true value. Further, it is comprised of the sum of the variance and squared bias of the estimator. These values were the basis of comparisons among the experimental designs.

In the one-drug study the dosage levels ranged from 0 to 1 unit, with the same fixed sample size of 48 observations for each design. The designs studied varied the intensity of the coverage of the treatment space versus the amount of replication of individual treatment points. Designs of 4, 8, and 24 equally spaced treatment points were considered. The replication factor of the 4-point design is therefore six times that of the 24-point scheme.

The size of the second design moment, $\Sigma_{i=1}^{N}(x_i - \bar{x})^2/N$, is important to the characterization of any design. Myers [6] indicates that designs with larger second moments have an advantage in their ability to view the surface over those designs with less spread. Thus, the designs considered in this study were all scaled to have equal second design moments while all treatment points were required to stay within the (0, 1) dosage interval. Once the design moments are equalized, the statistical evaluation of the different designs is possible. When faced with an actual design problem, however, the advantage of large second design moments must be considered.

The simulation study of combinations of two drugs was performed to assess the relative value of four designs performed on the unit square. Each of the four designs were evaluated for two response surfaces and two hazard functions. As each design consisted of 108 subjects, and as 300 repetitions of each situation were accomplished, 518,400 randomly generated survival times were used in the study.

Three of the designs investigated were 3^2, 6^2, and a rotatable central composite design. The factorial designs, prior to scaling, were composed of evenly spaced points including points on the edges of the experimental region. The central composite design before scaling was centered at (0.5, 0.5) with the axial points on the region's border. Each point in the 3^2 and the central composite was replicated 12 times, and the 6^2 was repeated three times. The fourth design was generated by augmenting the central composite with a treatment at each corner of the region. The addition of four center points to eight replications of this design required 108 sampling units, just as in the other three designs. Hereafter, the 108-point central composite design will be termed the CCD and the augmented one the ACCD. These designs were selected to compare designs found to be useful in a linear model situation

when fitting a quadratic response, namely the 3^2 or CCD, to
designs more commonly used in animal experiments. Each design
center is (0.5, 0.5) and the designs are all symmetric in X_1
and X_2. Scaling was such that all designs had the same vector
of second moments as the CCD. These designs are illustrated
in Fig. 5.2.

The conclusions of the simulation study follow. (Stablein
[7] gives, in tabular form, the data from which these conclusions are drawn.)

1. In one drug, increased density of treatment points is
   superior to extra replication of fewer treatments. The
   designs, ranked according to their estimation capabil-
   ities, show the 24-point to be superior to the 8-point,
   and the 8-point to be better than the 4-point. This
   finding appears to be independent of the level of
   censoring.

2. In two drugs, the 6^2 design was the best of those considered and the CCD the worst; the 3^2 and the ACCD were
   indistinguishable.

3. Differences in design appear to be unaffected by
   changing the underlying survival distributions.

4. Changing parameterizations produces no noticeable
   effects on relative design quality.

5. Extensive grouping of survival times causes the underestimation of the absolute magnitude of the model
   parameters, but does not affect relative design value.

These conclusions suggest that fixed resources should be
spread out among many treatment points. Further, providing that
the total sample is large enough, extensive replication of each
design point, contrary to present practice, is not necessary.
Thus, for example, it would appear possible to decrease the number of animals per treatment group in the three-drug design developed by Goldin et al. [4] and still have enough information
available to adequately describe the underlying treatment-
response surface.

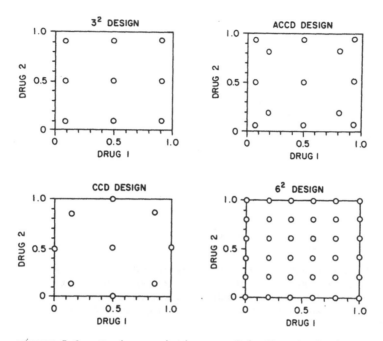

FIGURE 5.2. Design variations used in the simulation study: 3^2 and 6^2 = factorial designs; ACCD = augmented central composite design; CCD = central composite design.

Although important lessons have been learned through the simulation studies, problems remain in designing experiments which involve many variables. A four-drug factorial experiment with two individuals per group at five dosage levels requires 1250 individuals. (This would represent an expansion of the factorial design in Fig. 5.1B to four dimensions with only two individuals per point.) To accommodate the design for such experiments certain treatment groups must be omitted. However, when nothing is known about the nature of a response surface there is no basis for rationally omitting any treatment groups. When drug doses are the variables involved, certain reasonable assumptions can be made that are useful in defining the region of interest. If one considers a two-drug combination to be

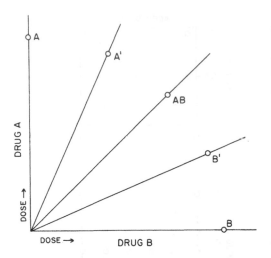

FIGURE 5.3. *Representation of the ridge of optimum responses.*
Points on the rays represent the optimum response for each
fixed dose-ratio treatment. Assuming an infinite number of
rays, the points would merge to form the ridge of optimum
responses.

represented graphically as shown in Fig. 5.3, with each fixed-
ratio drug treatment being considered as a single drug, one
would assume that as the dose increases, the effect increases
up to the optimum point and then decreases. Therefore, there
must be a ridge of optimum doses connecting the optimum dose
of drug A with the optimum dose of drug B.

Experiments done on a ray design support this contention.
The ridge of optimum values may bow in or out from a line connecting the optimum doses of the single drugs. A well-designed
experiment should include points in this region with points
falling on both sides of the ridge of optimum values. Little
is gained by adding many groups with ineffective treatments or
groups with highly lethal treatments.

In Fig. 5.1B, if the points only between F and F' or G and
G' are included, results are likely to be almost as satisfactory
as those of a full factorial experiment. Any knowledge of the

toxicity of even one combination of the drugs might help in
anticipating whether the ridge of optimum values bows in or out
to assist in selecting the FF' modification or the GG' modification. These modifications of the factorial design can easily
be adapted for use with three- or four-drug combinations and
result in considerably fewer treatment groups. The ratio of
the number of groups utilized to the number of groups on the
full factorial design drops as the number of drugs increases.
Experiments on these modified designs using up to four drugs
in combination are practical for use in the laboratory setting.

5.3 EFFECTS OF GROUPING ON CENSORED SURVIVAL DATA

In murine cancer chemotherapy survival experiments such as
those examples considered in previous chapters, the frequency
of survival assessment (which results in the grouping of otherwise distinct failure times), and the percentage of right-hand
single censoring are under experimental control. As such, they
become design variables, with both practical constraints and
statistical needs playing a role in their selection. Although
the practical constraints may be known, the effects of varying
grouping and censoring levels on the statistical analysis of
such experiments are not. Furthermore, in the proportional
hazard model, Eq. (3.7) is an approximation to the exact likelihood. Thus, it is important to evaluate the effect of this
approximation in such circumstances. As in the previous section, it is not possible to arrive at an analytic expression
which gives the properties of the parameter estimators as functions of censoring and grouping levels. Hence, a simulation
study is useful. Such a study was performed by Stablein and
Carter [8].

The simulations, performed to assess the statistical properties of the parameter estimates and estimates of optimal response, were modeled after advanced L1210 murine leukemia

chemotherapy experiments. As discussed earlier in this text,
the purpose of such experiments is to learn of the action of
the drug(s) and to determine optimal drug levels. Groups of
nearly identical animals receive treatments on predetermined
days after tumor injection, and the response of interest,
survival time, is checked at regular intervals. If treatment
begins seven days after tumor injection, then substantial numbers of deaths occur from both disease and toxicity soon after
treatment. As the control animals usually die within several
days of the treatment, the underlying survival distributions
were selected to have a mean of 2 time units. Two hazard functions that generate distributions from the Weibull family with
the mean of 2 were used. The first, a constant hazard $\lambda_o(t) =$
0.5, yields an exponential distribution with mean 2 and variance 4. A decreasing hazard function $\lambda_o(t) = 0.5t^{-0.5}$, imply-
ing a survival distribution with the same mean and variance of
20, provided a second situation for investigation.

In cancer chemotherapy applications it is reasonable to
expect the hazard function to decrease with increasing dosage
levels until the treatment's underlying toxicity equals its
beneficial effects. From this point on in the treatment space,
increases in drug levels will cause a rise in the hazard func-
tion. Using the reasoning previously outlined, $\underline{x}'\underline{\beta}$ was set
equal to a quadratic function in the dosage levels of the drugs
administered. It has been shown by Carter, Stablein, and
Wampler [2] to provide an adequate approximation of the actual
response surface.

In this study only a single drug was considered. Thus

$$\lambda(t) = \lambda_0(t) \ \exp(\beta_1 x + \beta_{11} x^2)$$

where x is the dose of the drug. Consistent with the results
of the previous section, the single design employed was composed of six evenly spaced points on the unit dose interval,

with eight subjects per experimental point. The dose-response surface parameters were selected to correspond to a relatively shallow treatment effect with the optimum near the center of the experimental region. Thus, $\underline{\beta}$ equaled (-4.54523, 3.72560) and x_{opt}, the treatment level with minimum relative hazard, equaled 0.61 while y_{opt}, the associated minimum response, was 0.25. Therefore, when $\lambda_o(t) = 0.5$ the distribution at the optimum has a mean of 8, and the median lifetime associated with x_{opt} is 5.55 as opposed to 1.39 when $x = 0.0$. For the long-tailed distribution the mean lifetime changes from 2 to 32 and the median from 0.48 to 7.69 when going from $x = 0.0$ to x_{opt}.

The probability integral transformation was used to generate the simulated failure times. To obtain grouped data, the authors let Δt represent the constant time interval between assessments of survival status. Deaths within the interval were recorded at the next time of assessment, so that if grouping occurred the observed t_j equaled $\Delta t [t_j / \Delta t]$, where [ ] is the next greatest integer function.

Each simulated experiment consisted of generating 48 failure times. Maximum-likelihood estimation of the parameters was accomplished with the Newton-Raphson technique. The estimated optimum dose $\hat{x}_{opt}$ was determined by algebraically maximizing the estimated relative hazard $\exp(\underline{x}'\hat{\underline{\beta}})$ with the restriction that the estimated optimum lie within the experimental region, while $\hat{y}_{opt}$, the estimated optimum response, was

$$\hat{y}_{opt} = \exp(\hat{\beta}_1 \hat{x}_{opt} + \hat{\beta}_{11} \hat{x}^2_{opt})$$

For each hazard function 400 sets of survival times, i.e., 400 experiments of size 48, were generated; each set was analyzed under all combinations of five right-hand censoring levels and four grouping structures. Censoring the largest 16, 10, 5, and 3 times corresponded to 33.3%, 20.83%, 10.42%, and 6.25%

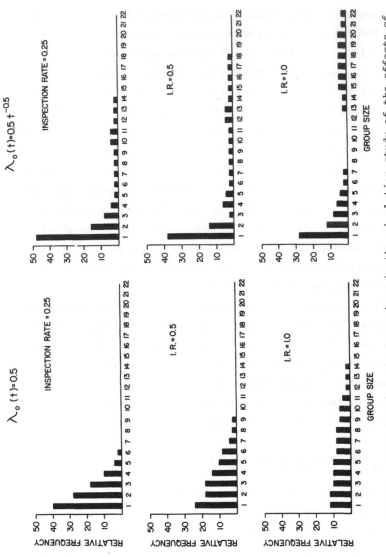

FIGURE 5.4. Distribution of group sizes in the simulation study of the effects of grouping on censored survival data. (From Ref. 8.)

censoring, respectively, while the fifth level was 0% censoring. Any additional observations grouped with those censored times were also censored. Data were analyzed without grouping, which yields the exact likelihood, and, alternatively, by assessing failure at every 0.25, 0.5, and 1 time unit. Thus, the effect of varying grouping and censoring levels was studied.

Figure 5.4 provides an indication of the number of nominally tied observations under the various grouping structures. It illustrates the average observed percentage of observations found in groups of given size. Notice that the patterns differ in that the distribution with constant hazard has fewer ungrouped observations as well as smaller sets of tied survival times. Even when the survival experience is assessed four times every time unit, over one-half of the observations do not have distinct failure times. Further, when $\Delta t = 1$ an average of 15 distinct failure times are observed. Note also that the single right-censoring pattern employed will result in even fewer distinct failure times, as long-term survivors will be censored.

Tables 5.1 and 5.2 contain estimated median efficiencies and associated approximate 95% confidence limits for the statistics $\hat{\beta}_1$, $\hat{\beta}_{11}$, $\hat{x}_{opt}$, and $\hat{y}_{opt}$. Efficiency is defined for a given simulated experiment as the ratio of the reciprocal of the mean square error for a given-group censoring level to the corresponding reciprocal mean square error for the ungrouped, 0% censoring analysis. Efficiencies exceeding unity indicate improved relative performance.

Examining first the efficiency of the estimation of β_1 and β_{11}, one notes significant increases in efficiency associated with slight grouping and censoring in both distributions. For example, with the constant hazard function $\Delta t = 0.25$ and 6.25% censoring, the median efficiency of $\hat{\beta}_1$ is 1.096 and its 95% confidence interval ranges from 1.031 to 1.135. Similar improvements are found with the decreasing hazard function at these levels. Efficiencies in excess of 1, as regards $\hat{y}_{opt}$,

TABLE 5.1. Median Efficiencies and 95% Confidence Intervals for the Estimation of Parameters and Optima for Various Grouping and Censoring Levels for $\lambda_0(t) = 0.5$

Grouping interval Δt		Censoring level				
		0%	6.25%	10.42%	20.83%	33.33%
0	$\hat{\beta}_1$	1.000	1.000 (0.981, 1.000)	0.967 (0.934, 1.006)	0.940 (0.859, 1.024)	0.784 (0.694, 0.904)
	$\hat{\beta}_{11}$	1.000	1.000 (1.000, 1.000)	0.974 (0.935, 1.005)	0.903 (0.795, 0.971)	0.761 (0.676, 0.890)
	$\hat{x}_{opt}$	1.000	1.000 (0.986, 1.000)	0.956 (0.887, 1.000)	0.901 (0.799, 0.961)	0.779 (0.655, 0.932)
	$\hat{y}_{opt}$	1.000	1.000 (1.000, 1.003)	0.989 (0.963, 1.009)	1.026 (0.965, 1.083)	0.957 (0.884, 1.018)
0.25	$\hat{\beta}_1$	1.040 (0.988, 1.080)	1.096 (1.031, 1.135)	1.047 (0.976, 1.140)	1.074 (1.000, 1.182)	0.858 (0.740, 0.978)
	$\hat{\beta}_{11}$	1.053 (1.014, 1.081)	1.079 (1.030, 1.119)	1.073 (0.976, 1.125)	1.015 (0.900, 1.103)	0.828 (0.736, 0.978)
	$\hat{x}_{opt}$	0.996 (0.974, 1.002)	0.970 (0.935, 1.000)	0.962 (0.876, 1.000)	0.858 (0.772, 0.970)	0.776 (0.644, 0.923)
	$\hat{y}_{opt}$	1.034 (0.975, 1.070)	1.080 (1.031, 1.117)	1.063 (0.982, 1.086)	1.124 (1.041, 1.181)	0.991 (0.906, 1.070)
0.5	$\hat{\beta}_1$	1.009 (0.936, 1.259)	1.195 (1.026, 1.304)	1.164 (0.989, 1.292)	1.099 (1.000, 1.316)	0.969 (0.802, 1.190)
	$\hat{\beta}_{11}$	1.089 (1.000, 1.235)	1.199 (1.093, 1.328)	1.166 (1.030, 1.292)	1.126 (0.965, 1.244)	0.910 (0.740, 1.120)
	$\hat{x}_{opt}$	0.966 (0.936, 1.000)	0.951 (0.903, 1.000)	0.917 (0.847, 0.995)	0.874 (0.797, 0.960)	0.745 (0.610, 0.858)
	$\hat{y}_{opt}$	0.991 (0.843, 1.181)	1.120 (0.943, 1.239)	1.117 (1.005, 1.202)	1.183 (1.045, 1.261)	1.016 (0.923, 1.189)
1	$\hat{\beta}_1$	0.811 (0.736, 0.980)	1.021 (0.864, 1.431)	1.059 (0.855, 1.504)	1.139 (0.837, 1.495)	0.980 (0.784, 1.241)
	$\hat{\beta}_{11}$	0.887 (0.778, 1.059)	1.157 (0.960, 1.550)	1.227 (0.910, 1.527)	1.167 (0.898, 1.330)	0.964 (0.742, 1.190)
	$\hat{x}_{opt}$	0.952 (0.901, 0.992)	0.948 (0.876, 0.993)	0.923 (0.838, 1.000)	0.842 (0.724, 0.896)	0.776 (0.612, 0.860)
	$\hat{y}_{opt}$	0.675 (0.584, 0.822)	0.899 (0.718, 1.471)	0.956 (0.755, 1.416)	1.024 (0.772, 1.391)	0.952 (0.810, 1.312)

Source: Ref. 8.

TABLE 5.2. *Median Efficiencies and 95% Confidence Intervals for the Estimation of Parameters and Optima for Various Grouping and Censoring Levels for* $\lambda_0(t) = 0.5t^{-0.5}$

Grouping interval Δt		Censoring level				
		0%	6.25%	10.42%	20.83%	33.33%
0	$\hat{\beta}_1$	1.000	1.000 (0.993, 1.010)	1.021 (0.981, 1.062)	0.906 (0.826, 0.987)	0.843 (0.731, 0.928)
	$\hat{\beta}_{11}$	1.000	1.000 (1.000, 1.009)	1.019 (0.996, 1.076)	0.912 (0.826, 1.001)	0.813 (0.703, 0.953)
	$\hat{x}_{opt}$	1.000	1.000 (0.992, 1.012)	0.994 (0.966, 1.038)	0.867 (0.777, 0.954)	0.738 (0.646, 0.879)
	$\hat{y}_{opt}$	1.000	1.000 (0.993, 1.002)	1.011 (0.986, 1.037)	0.989 (0.923, 1.035)	0.920 (0.842, 0.983)
0.25	$\hat{\beta}_1$	1.122 (1.019, 1.230)	1.195 (1.060, 1.269)	1.271 (1.167, 1.342)	1.110 (0.952, 1.227)	0.998 (0.797, 1.195)
	$\hat{\beta}_{11}$	1.114 (1.034, 1.196)	1.185 (1.066, 1.236)	1.221 (1.149, 1.325)	1.020 (0.903, 1.121)	0.894 (0.732, 1.103)
	$\hat{x}_{opt}$	0.966 (0.938, 0.988)	0.982 (0.946, 1.017)	0.962 (0.859, 1.018)	0.858 (0.781, 0.912)	0.721 (0.590, 0.887)
	$\hat{y}_{opt}$	1.153 (1.049, 1.255)	1.205 (1.100, 1.285)	1.203 (1.117, 1.289)	1.153 (1.057, 1.250)	1.038 (0.907, 1.193)
0.5	$\hat{\beta}_1$	1.070 (0.925, 1.406)	1.155 (0.967, 1.447)	1.252 (1.066, 1.439)	1.222 (0.980, 1.383)	0.962 (0.784, 1.193)
	$\hat{\beta}_{11}$	1.153 (0.971, 1.330)	1.222 (1.033, 1.362)	1.328 (1.156, 1.511)	1.139 (0.967, 1.294)	0.963 (0.782, 1.182)
	$\hat{x}_{opt}$	0.951 (0.916, 0.978)	0.964 (0.898, 1.008)	0.926 (0.840, 0.981)	0.833 (0.750, 0.980)	0.698 (0.585, 0.861)
	$\hat{y}_{opt}$	1.100 (0.923, 1.350)	1.182 (0.958, 1.404)	1.212 (1.053, 1.458)	1.229 (1.060, 1.412)	1.034 (0.845, 1.253)
1	$\hat{\beta}_1$	0.884 (0.781, 1.255)	0.898 (0.754, 1.361)	0.966 (0.792, 1.307)	0.938 (0.754, 1.182)	0.702 (0.556, 0.907)
	$\hat{\beta}_{11}$	1.025 (0.882, 1.495)	1.049 (0.906, 1.418)	1.247 (0.990, 1.499)	1.119 (0.884, 1.497)	0.868 (0.633, 1.106)
	$\hat{x}_{opt}$	0.926 (0.881, 0.973)	0.917 (0.855, 1.000)	0.895 (0.888, 0.959)	0.766 (0.689, 0.857)	0.673 (0.542, 0.779)
	$\hat{y}_{opt}$	0.760 (0.671, 0.929)	0.816 (0.693, 0.991)	0.808 (0.722, 1.174)	0.909 (0.642, 1.144)	0.706 (0.545, 1.053)

Source: Ref. 8.

are also evident when moderately grouped data are not exten-
sively censored. Deterioration in the median efficiency of
estimation of parameters and of y_{opt} is noted with increased
Δt or percent censoring, but the decreases are seldom significant. One notes instead increasingly wider confidence intervals, with widths in excess of 0.5 not being uncommon when
$\Delta t = 1$.

The effects of varying grouping and censoring levels on
the estimated optimum dose have none of the unusual character-
istics associated with the other statistics. In many situations, significantly decreased efficiency in the estimation of
the optimum result. The observed deterioration appears to be
affected more by increased censoring for fixed Δt than by increased grouping for fixed censoring percentage in the ranges
considered. Likewise, the associated confidence intervals
appear to be narrower and more stable than those of other
statistics.

In Tables 5.3 and 5.4 the average percent bias and associated standard errors are reported. For both distributions the
parameters are significantly positively biased. When no grouping of the data occurs, as Δt increases, the bias is eliminated
and then becomes significantly negative. The effect of censoring on this bias is negligible. The estimate of the response
for the optimum, $\hat{y}_{opt}$, is unbiased at $\Delta t = 0$, but it is also
substantially affected by increased grouping. In fact, with
$\Delta t = 1$ serious positive bias causes underestimation of the effectiveness of the treatment in the decreasing hazard function.
The estimate of x_{opt} performs much better as regards bias.
Neither grouping nor censoring has an important effect on the
bias of $\hat{x}_{opt}$, which remains small and positive throughout the
table. Thus, although the variability $\hat{x}_{opt}$ increases with
grouping and censoring, its bias remains nearly unchanged from
that observed in the complete information situation.

TABLE 5.3. *Effects of Grouping and Censoring on the Percentage of Bias in Parameter Estimates and Optima for* $\lambda_0(t) = 0.5$

Grouping interval Δt		Censoring level									
		0%		6.25%		10.42%		20.83%		33.33%	
		% Bias	SE	% Bias	SE	% Bias	SE	% Bias	SE	% Bias	SE
0	$\hat{\beta}_1$	6.618	2.00	6.655	2.00	6.237	2.04	4.840	2.12	3.238	2.23
	$\hat{\beta}_{11}$	7.140	2.27	7.256	2.28	6.708	2.33	4.823	2.45	2.916	2.59
	$\hat{x}_{opt}$	3.464	0.86	3.403	0.86	3.863	0.90	5.245	1.00	6.149	1.07
	$\hat{y}_{opt}$	1.437	2.49	1.400	2.46	1.734	2.47	2.514	2.54	4.997	2.77
0.25	$\hat{\beta}_1$	1.118	1.99	2.960	1.92	2.472	1.96	1.143	2.02	0.605	2.14
	$\hat{\beta}_{11}$	1.799	2.24	3.620	2.20	2.988	2.25	1.150	2.36	0.884	2.51
	$\hat{x}_{opt}$	3.181	0.93	3.411	0.88	3.829	0.91	5.327	1.02	6.341	1.09
	$\hat{y}_{opt}$	9.916	2.80	5.684	2.46	6.127	2.48	6.550	2.52	9.281	2.77
0.5	$\hat{\beta}_1$	-4.713	2.02	-0.813	1.83	-1.296	1.87	-2.276	1.93	-4.522	2.05
	$\hat{\beta}_{11}$	-3.817	2.25	-0.074	2.11	-0.691	2.16	-2.111	2.26	-4.743	2.42
	$\hat{x}_{opt}$	3.087	0.98	3.288	0.87	3.742	0.91	5.145	1.02	6.539	1.11
	$\hat{y}_{opt}$	20.300	3.23	10.477	2.48	10.910	2.51	10.983	2.54	14.185	2.79
1	$\hat{\beta}_1$	-15.361	1.95	-7.729	1.70	-8.207	1.74	-9.409	1.80	-11.293	1.93
	$\hat{\beta}_{11}$	-14.194	2.16	-6.903	1.98	-7.492	2.04	-9.305	2.14	-11.394	2.30
	$\hat{x}_{opt}$	2.809	1.04	3.290	0.87	3.732	0.91	5.445	1.04	6.823	1.15
	$\hat{y}_{opt}$	39.090	3.61	20.181	2.52	20.568	2.55	20.983	2.60	23.703	2.85

Source: Ref. 8.

TABLE 5.4. Effects of Grouping and Censoring on the Percentage of Bias in Parameter Estimates and Optima for $\lambda_0(t) = 0.5t^{-0.5}$

Grouping interval Δt		Censoring level								
		0%		6.25%		10.42%		20.83%		33.33%
		% Bias	SE	% Bias	SE	% Bias	SE	% Bias	SE	% Bias	SE
0	$\hat{\beta}_1$	7.861	1.96	7.536	1.96	7.347	1.96	6.144	2.06	4.194	2.19
	$\hat{\beta}_{11}$	9.743	2.33	9.348	2.33	8.971	2.33	7.544	2.48	5.314	2.62
	$\hat{x}_{opt}$	2.465	0.83	2.496	0.83	2.815	0.85	3.759	0.94	4.205	1.00
	$\hat{y}_{opt}$	-0.010	2.29	0.374	2.33	0.236	2.31	1.542	2.45	4.642	2.71
0.25	$\hat{\beta}_1$	0.788	1.83	0.648	1.82	0.433	1.81	-1.046	1.81	-3.408	2.04
	$\hat{\beta}_{11}$	2.902	2.22	2.662	2.21	2.273	2.20	0.539	2.20	-2.170	2.48
	$\hat{x}_{opt}$	2.542	0.86	2.533	0.86	2.672	0.85	3.750	0.85	4.259	1.03
	$\hat{y}_{opt}$	8.840	2.35	8.596	2.30	8.560	2.28	10.285	2.28	13.828	2.72
0.5	$\hat{\beta}_1$	-3.438	1.75	-3.616	1.74	-3.849	1.73	-5.428	1.82	-8.040	1.94
	$\hat{\beta}_{11}$	-1.172	2.14	-1.452	2.13	-1.854	2.12	-3.704	2.26	-6.666	2.39
	$\hat{x}_{opt}$	2.413	0.87	2.468	0.88	2.578	0.86	3.705	0.98	4.507	1.07
	$\hat{y}_{opt}$	14.521	2.33	14.352	2.29	14.391	2.27	16.217	2.44	20.277	2.72
1	$\hat{\beta}_1$	-10.386	1.65	-10.312	1.63	-10.528	1.62	-12.213	1.71	-15.519	1.09
	$\hat{\beta}_{11}$	-7.996	2.03	-8.044	2.02	-8.416	2.01	-10.374	2.14	-14.102	1.53
	$\hat{x}_{opt}$	2.355	0.89	2.460	0.90	2.573	0.88	3.524	0.98	4.455	0.64
	$\hat{y}_{opt}$	25.089	2.38	24.282	2.29	24.312	2.27	26.423	2.45	32.111	2.81

Source: Ref. 8.

REFERENCES

1. Box, G. E. P., and Wilson, K. B. (1951). On the experimental attainment of optimum conditions. *J. Roy. Stat. Soc. B, 13*, 1–45.

2. Carter, W. H., Jr., Stablein, D. M., and Wampler, G. L. (1979). An improved method for analyzing survival data from combination chemotherapy experiments. *Cancer Res., 39*, 3446–3453.

3. Goldin, A., Venditti, J. M., Humphreys, S. R., and Mantel, N. (1956). Modification of treatment schedules in the management of advanced mouse leukemia with amethopterin. *J. Nat. Cancer Inst., 17*, 203–212.

4. Goldin, A., Venditti, J. M., Mantel, N., Kline, I., and Gang, M. (1968). Evaluation of combination chemotherapy with three drugs. *Cancer Res., 28*, 950–961.

5. Mantel, N. (1958). An experimental design in combination chemotherapy. *Ann. N.Y. Acad. Sci., 76*, 909–931.

6. Myers, R. H. (1976). Response surface methodology. Department of Statistics, Virginia Polytechnic Institute and State University, Blacksburg.

7. Stablein, D. M. (1979). Design and analysis of combination chemotherapy survival experiments. Unpublished doctoral dissertation, Medical College of Virginia, Virginia Commonwealth University, Richmond.

8. Stablein, D. M., and Carter, W. H., Jr. (1980). A Monte Carlo study of the effects of grouping on the analysis of censored survival data. *J. Stat. Comp. and Simul., 14*, 113–123.

9. Venditti, J. M., Humphreys, S. R., Mantel, N., and Goldin, A. (1956). Combined treatment of advanced leukemia (L-1210) in mice using amethopterin and 6-mercaptopurine. *J. Nat. Cancer Inst., 17*, 631–638.

10. Wampler, G. L., Carter, W. H., Jr., and Williams, V. R. (1978). Combination chemotherapy: Arriving at optimal treatment levels by incorporating side effect constraints. *Cancer Treat. Rep., 62*, 333–340.

6

Interpretation of Analytic Results

6.1 INTRODUCTION

With a knowledge of the response surface associated with a combination of drugs, it is possible to gain an understanding of how the drugs can be used together optimally. For example, a more fundamental knowledge of the properties of the drugs involved may be gained as a result of the information contained in the response surface which relates to the manner in which the drugs interact. Such information might lead to a modification of the use of the given combination by suggesting a decrease in the dosage of one or more of the drugs and an increase in the dosages of the remaining drugs.

Since the underlying response surface is not likely to be known, it is necessary to estimate and explore it using the techniques discussed in the preceding chapters. It is the intent of this chapter to discuss the interpretation of such statistical analyses by means of examples involving the use of drug combinations in animal models. The extent to which the knowledge of dose response surfaces in animals will help in optimizing combination treatments in man is not yet known. At the very least, the experiments in animals will provide knowledge of how optimization experiments might reasonably be conducted in humans.

6.2 RELATIONSHIP OF SURVIVAL TO TUMOR CELL KILL

A relationship exists between tumor cell kill by chemotherapeutic agents and dose-survival response curves or surfaces.
This relationship needs to be explored in order to best under-
stand the surfaces that will be presented.

Chemotherapeutic agents are known to kill both normal and
malignant cells as a function of dose. The type of cell-kill
curve observed varies with the drug, but many drugs kill cells
in a manner similar to radiation. Until a threshold dose is
attained few cells are killed. Then as the dose increases
arithmetically, cell kill increases exponentially. The plotted
(semilog) cell-kill curve consists of a shoulder region in the
subthreshold dosage range, followed by a linear component. The
size of the shoulder region is related to the capacity of
treated cells to repair sublethal damage. Differences in shoulder size and the rates of repair among various normal and neoplastic cells may greatly influence the optimal schedule of
treatments [6]. The slope of the linear component is related
to the relative sensitivity of the cells to the agent utilized.
As neoplastic cells become resistant to treatment the slope
changes, although the shoulder region and extrapolation number
do not [4]. Upward concavities in the linear component of the
dose-survival response curve (changes in slope after a certain
fractional cell kill) indicate subpopulations of cells with
less drug sensitivity. There is a slight upward concavity in
the exponential portion of the response of L1210 cells to cyclophosphamide (CTX) treatment, indicating that a small subpopula-
tion ($\cong$ 2%) of cells is slightly more resistant than the remainder [4, 5]. Cell kill curves for cell-cycle phase-specific drugs,
e.g., hydroxyurea [2], may become horizontal after all vulner-
able cells are killed, indicating that cells not in a specific
phase are completely insensitive to drug action.

DeWys has provided data on L1210 cell kill with CTX treatment by doing serial counts of ascites cells after administering various doses of CTX [5]. Using these data and assuming a doubling time of 12 hr and death of the animal after the total cell count exceeds 10^{10} cells, one can construct dose response curves for various treatment regimens. Figure 6.1 demonstrates calculated and experimental dose response curves for CTX given on a daily schedule. The correspondence of the curves indicates that, as one might surmise, the dose response can be related to cell kill at least in the initial region of the response curve shown in Fig. 6.1. The shoulder region discussed above is also very much in evidence on the survival plot.

At higher doses, dose-survival response curves calculated from cell-kill information fail because of host toxicity. Comparison of dose-survival response curves of tumor-bearing and nontumor-bearing animals indicates that the major contributing factor in the descending aspect of such plots is drug-induced

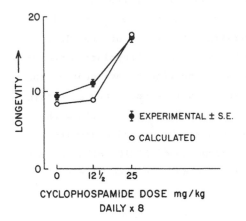

FIGURE 6.1. Observed and calculated survival of mice bearing L1210 leukemia with daily cyclophosphamide treatment. Calculation was made using cell-kill information and L1210 kinetic data.

host lethality [12].   In fact, a reasonable representation of a
dose-survival response curve can be obtained by combining the
independently obtained results of cell-kill and host-lethality
data as shown in the dotted line in Fig. 6.2.   The actual dose-
survival response curve lies below the calculated one.   Multiple factors both known and unknown contribute to this phenome-
non.   In the example above the cell-kill information was
obtained from ascites cells subjected to in vivo treatment.
Schenken has shown that metastatic P815x2 tumor cells are more

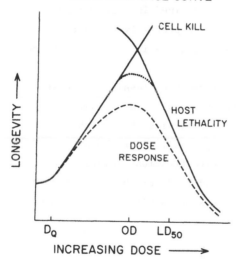

ANALYSIS OF COMPONENTS OF
DOSE RESPONSE CURVE

D_Q = Quasi-threshold dose
OD = Optimal dose
LD_{50} = Lethal dose 50% of animal

FIGURE 6.2.   *Analysis of components of a dose response curve.*
Dots = additive result of combining cell-kill and host-
lethality curves
Dashes = observed curve
D_0 = quasi threshold dose
OD = optimal dose
LD_{50} = lethal dose to 50% of animals

resistant than ascites cells to treatment with 1,3-bis(2-chloro-
ethyl)-1-nitrosourea (BCNU), while solid tumors are still more
refractory to BCNU [10]. Multiple investigators have shown that
dividing and nondividing cells have differing sensitivities to
treatments [1, 10, 11]. The proportion of dividing and nondividing cells changes with age of the tumor and likely also with
the site and size of metastasis. Obviously, tumor cells that
have migrated to sanctuary areas are more resistant to treatment. This is because of poor drug penetration into the tissue.
A spectrum of different drug levels in different tissues (shown
very nicely with radioactive doxorubicin in the rat [7]), obviously results in different sensitivities to treatment. For these
reasons, the cell-kill information obtained in vitro or in a
single tissue could not be expected to precisely reflect host
survival and would likely be least accurate in advanced disease
states.

Up to this point we have explored the classical dose-survival response curve where longevity is plotted by dose of
drug(s) given. It is important to recognize that in the models
that have been developed either a probability or the natural
logarithm of the risk associated with treatment relative to
that of the control group is plotted by dose; the form of such
functions may not be precisely the same as with survival curves
or surfaces.

6.3 INTERPRETATION OF CONTOUR PLOTS

The contour plots for a combination of k drugs are plots of
constant response (relative hazard or probability of favorable
outcome, depending on the analysis) for all possible combinations of two drugs within a given range of doses. If more than
two drugs have been tested in the combination, plots can be generated for all possible two-drug combinations at fixed levels
of all other drugs in the combination. By considering multiple

levels of the other drugs, a reasonable impression of the relationships which exist between all drugs in the combination can be gained. The contour plots are constructed so that the regions of the treatment space associated with better treatment are indicated by progressively darker shading.

The interpretation of contours of constant response which result from a logistic regression analysis is straightforward, and there is no difficulty in comparing regions of optimal treatment from experiment to experiment. However, when one compares contour plots of the relative hazard functions care must be exercised. From the definition of terms in the statistical model it is apparent that $\exp(\underline{x}'\underline{\hat{\beta}})$, the relative hazard function and the quantity plotted, is the ratio of the hazard function associated with treatment condition $\underline{x}$ to the hazard function associated with the control groups. Therefore, the different shadings of the contour plots indicate regions in the treatment space where the hazard is a multiple (usually a fractional value) of that of the control group. Since $\lambda_0(t)$, the hazard function associated with the control groups, is never specified, it follows that the shadings associated with the various regions on the contour plots from experiment to experiment should not be compared unless one is willing to assume equality of the hazards associated with the control groups. In general, hazard-function plots for P388 leukemia have lighter shading (higher relative hazard) than for L1210 leukemia, even though the animals have a lower absolute hazard, i.e., they live longer than animals with L1210 leukemia. (Compare Figs. 6.3A and B to 6.3C and D, and Figs. 6.4A and B to 6.4C and D.) This has been attributed to the fact that the variance of the survival distribution of control animals with L1210 leukemia appears to be less than that of control animals with P388 leukemia. Thus, identical relative hazards from different experiments may have different meanings.

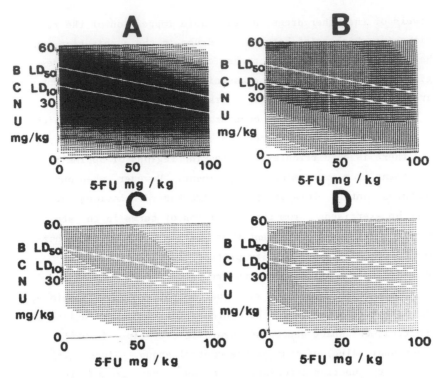

FIGURE 6.3.   *Dose-relative hazard response surfaces for com-bination of 5-fluorouracil and BCNU.   (A, B)   Advanced L1210 leukemia; (C, D) advanced P388 leukemia with overlay of LD$_{10}$ and LD$_{50}$ values obtained from a logistic analysis of data from a separate experiment conducted in nontumored mice and duplicated in each panel.   All mice were B6D2F$_1$ female mice weighing 19 to 23 g.   Ten million tumor cells were inoculated s.c. (A and B) or i.p. (C and D) to establish the respective tumors.   Treatment was given as a single intraperitoneal in-jection of each drug on day 7.   Each panel represents a single experiment comprised of 16 treatment groups with eight animals per group.*

The contour lines represent isobols of constant response (equal biologic effect lines). Bisection of the geometric de-sign along the axis most nearly parallel to the line or plane through the optimum doses of the single drugs will give an approximation of the ridge of the optimum response, a

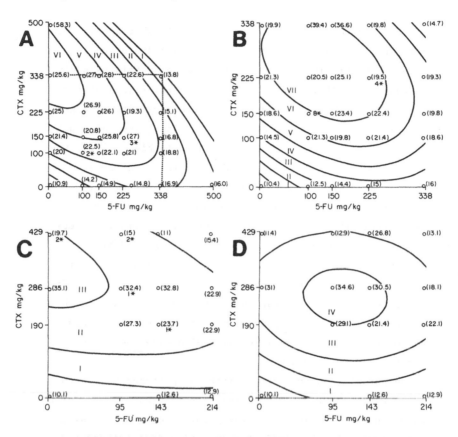

FIGURE 6.4.   *Dose-relative hazard response surfaces for combination of 5-fluorouracil and cyclophosphamide.   (A, B)   Advanced
L1210 leukemia;   (C, D) advanced P388 leukemia.*

  *Treatment was given by single intraperitoneal injection of
drugs.   For A and C drugs were given together on day 7 after
10⁶ leukemia cells on day 0; for B and D, 5-FU was given on day
7, 24 hr before CTX was given on day 8.   Roman numerals label
the different density zones of decreasing hazard.   Experimental
points are noted by the open dots with the corresponding mean
survival of mice shown in parentheses.   The number of survivors
is shown by an asterisk.   Survivors were not included in the
mean survival calculation.   Note the difference in scaling.
The dotted lines in A include the area shown in B.   Therapeutic
synergism, not evident when the drugs are administered simultaneously, is present when 5-FU is given 24 hr before CTX in both
advanced murine leukemias.*

hypothetical surface consisting of the n points of optimum response for n constant-ratio drug combinations discussed in
Chap. 5. Contour lines on the ordinate side of this axis give
an approximation of isobols of tumor cell kill (lines of equal
tumor cell kill) while contour lines on the opposite side give
an approximation of isobols of host lethality (lines of equal
lethality). These relationships are shown in Fig. 6.5 for the
combination of 5-fluorouracil (5-FU) and cisplatin (DDP), which
has been tested in both L1210 and P388 murine leukemias. Due
to the form of the model used, the contours are symmetrical.
It is unlikely that this is the situation in reality. Experiments conducted in therapeutic dosage ranges should better
represent isobols of tumor cell kill than isobols of toxicity.
The contours in the toxic area of the treatment space may often
be estimated to be wider than they actually are, based on the
knowledge that the toxicity of many chemotherapeutic agents
increases rapidly with small incremental dosage increases,
once a toxic dose is reached.

Contour plots with several different patterns have been
encountered in the two-drug combinations that have been analyzed
in this manner. One may encounter parallel contour lines. If
they are vertical, this indicates an active drug represented on
the abscissa and an inactive drug on the ordinate with no drug
interaction. An example is the vincristine/cyclophosphamide
experiment represented in Fig. 6.6. Parallel lines with a slope
of -1, assuming that the scaling from 0 to optimum dose is equal
for the two drugs, would indicate two equally active drugs with
no interaction effect. Slopes less than or greater than -1
under the same assumption would be seen with drugs of different
activity.

It would appear that closed surfaces are formed in situations in which favorable interactions are seen. Examples are

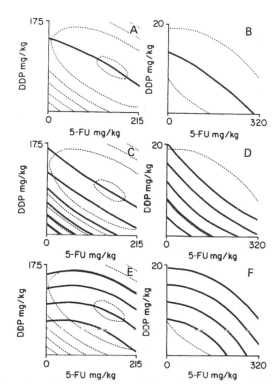

FIGURE 6.5. *Dose-relative hazard response surfaces for the combination of 5-fluorouracil (5-FU) and cisplatin (DDP).*
(A) Plots of the surface resulting from the analysis of data obtained from treatment of advanced L1210 leukemia. Dotted lines represent isobols of decreasing hazard with increasing dose up to the solid line overlay, which is assumed to be a representation of the ridge of optimum doses for fixed dose ratios of the two drugs. (B) A similar representation from data obtained from treatment of advanced P388 leukemia (note the difference in scaling). (C) Using the same L1210 data as for A, the solid overlay lines are assumed to be an approximation of isobols of tumor cell kill for the various combinations. (D) Isobols of tumor cell kill assumed for P388 leukemia. (E) Isobols of host lethality assumed from the L1210 data. (F) Isobols of host lethality assumed from the P388 data.

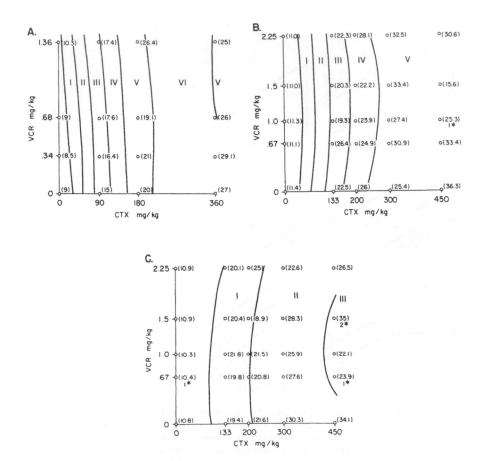

FIGURE 6.6. Dose-relative hazard response surface for combinations of vincristine and cyclophosphamide. (A) Advanced ascitic L1210; (B, C) advanced solid L1210 leukemia.

Drugs were given together in (A) and (B); cyclophosphamide was given 24 hr after vincristine in (C). Roman numerals label the different density zones of decreasing hazard. Experimental points are indicated by open dots, with the mean survival of the mice in each group shown in parentheses. The number of 100-day survivors is shown and denoted by an asterisk. Survivors were not included in the mean survival calculation. Cyclophosphamide, the active drug, was given on day 6, 7, and 8 after tumor inoculation in experiments represented by panels A, B, and C, respectively. This may in part be responsible for the differences in relative hazard seen. No interaction effect is apparent.

5-fluorouracil/cisplatin (Fig. 6.5) and 5-fluorouracil/cyclo-
phosphamide, more particularly when the 5-fluorouracil is given
24 hr before the cyclophosphamide (Fig. 6.4). For drugs with
low activity and flat dose response surfaces, e.g., cell-cycle
phase-specific agents given in a single dose, it is possible
that the estimated relationship will indicate that both low and

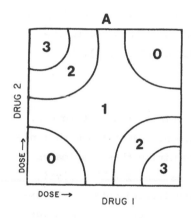

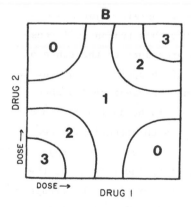

FIGURE 6.7. *These constructed response surfaces represent (A)*
what might be expected if an adverse interaction is seen with
two drugs with essentially equal activity and (B) an artifact
secondary to poor data. In each figure the higher numbers
indicate lower hazard.

high doses are better than therapeutic doses. Such a result is
obviously a distortion secondary to inadequate data or variability in the data and can be easily recognized, as a saddle system is produced in the plotted surfaces. However, not all saddle systems that are generated are artifacts. An example of a
true saddle system would occur when two drugs of essentially
equal activities have adverse interaction effects such that all
combination treatments are inferior to the optimum results of
either individual drug, as shown in Fig. 6.7A. The shading of
the zones would differ in this situation as compared to the
case where an artifact has been produced (Fig. 6.7B).

6.4 OPTIMUM DOSES

It is often of interest to estimate optimal treatment levels,
that is to define the levels of treatment associated with minimum estimated risk. Methods for determining these estimates
have been presented in the chapters describing each analytic
procedure. Any optimum doses that are located outside the experimental region are possibly invalid, since the formulation
for the dose response surfaces may well contain major distor-
tions outside the treatment field. For this reason it is cus-
tomary to constrain the optimization procedure to the range of
doses used in the experiment. Thus, if an optimal treatment is
estimated to be on the boundary of the treatment region when
such constraints are used, it is likely to be an indication of
an improperly chosen dosage range. In such situations a new
experiment should be performed in the range of dosages suggested by the analysis. When interpreting the results of the
optimization analysis it is necessary to correlate the findings
with the contour plots, since it is possible for the optimization procedure to converge at an inappropriate value. If this
should occur, repeating the procedure from a different starting
point usually leads to the correct result.

Extrapolation of animal optimum dose data to human treatment has not proven to be useful, probably because the relative
potency of drugs in the treatment of animal tumors differs from
their potency in treating human tumors; this undoubtedly influ-
ences the proportions of drugs that should be used in a combination. The relationships that exist between the drugs in a combination, as presented in the estimated response surface, contain information that more likely can be used to advantage in
the development of better treatments.

6.5 RELATIONSHIPS TO CLASSICAL DEFINITIONS OF DRUG INTERACTION

In order to treat cancer effectively with combinations of drugs,
it is important to describe and quantitate the types of interactions that occur. Historically, the terms synergism and
antagonism have been developed to define drug interactions.
These terms are best applied to situations in which the drug
effect continues to increase as the dose increases. In such
situations, if the drug-combination effect is greater than that
expected, on additive (or multiplicative) grounds, then the
term synergism is applied. If it is less than expected, the
term antagonism is applied.

Isobolograms have been utilized to graphically define drug
interactions [9] (Fig. 6.8). Isobiologic effect lines (isobols)
bowing toward the ordinate indicate synergism, while isobols
bowing away from the ordinate represent antagonism. It is important to recognize that the contour plots (Sect. 6.3) are
isobolograms and that contour lines representing synergism and
antagonism often appear on the same isobologram. This situation can occur because the effectiveness of any cytotoxic drug
or fixed-ratio combination of drugs eventually decreases beyond
an optimum dose, resulting in an equally effective dose on both
sides of the optimum. The isobols containing these points of
equal effect often have different configurations.

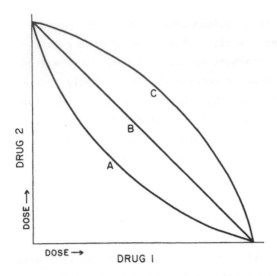

FIGURE 6.8. *Isobols of constant biologic effect.*
A = synergism
B = additivity
C = antagonism

The term therapeutic synergism was introduced by Venditti
et al. [13] to describe a situation in which the optimum result
obtained with a combination exceeded that which could be obtained with either drug used alone. This definition is one of
the more useful ones introduced but is somewhat deficient both
in quantifying the degrees of interaction seen and in describing the many patterns of interaction that most certainly exist.
The method used to experimentally demonstrate such a synergism
actually involves the comparison of only one group of animals
receiving a combination of drugs or combined modality treatment
with only one other group of animals receiving a single agent
or modality. The groups being compared are those giving the
most favorable response in the respective categories. It is
obvious that such a method ignores considerable useful information from an experiment. When therapeutic synergism is present the highest densities on the contour plots occur away from

the coordinate axes. The strength of the therapeutic synergism
is indicated by the difference in the shading at the optimum
dose and the maximum shading on any of the coordinate axes.
Since the contours are arbitrarily chosen, a more precise definition of therapeutic synergism has been developed by considering the confidence region about the optimal treatment level [3].

6.6 DUAL OR MULTIPLE RESPONSE SURFACES

The discussions and results presented up to now make it clear
that doses administered at a toxic level are necessary in order
to accurately model the underlying dose response surface. In
life-span data the toxicity involved is host lethality. Adequate experiments for estimation of dose-survival time response
surfaces require some host lethality. Obviously, some adapta-
tion of the methods will be required for human experimentation.

It is possible to use sublethal toxicity such as weight
loss, leukopenia, or thrombocytopenia in lieu of host lethality
by employing the techniques for dual or multiple response systems [8, 15]. By this method a sublethal toxicity that can be
conveniently measured and which is correlated with host lethality is used as a constraint on doses in the lethal range. Consider the hypothetical data in Table 6.1. Assuming that treatment of 100 subjects with combinations A/B results in nadir

*TABLE 6.1. Hypothetical Lethality
Secondary to Leukopenia*

Nadir (WBC/mm^3)	Lethality (%)
3000	0
1000 to 2999	0
500 to 999	2
100 to 499	10

counts down to 500 WBC/mm^3, with 10 patients in the 500 to 1000 range the expected lethality would be 0.2 patients. Isobols of WBC levels could be accurately constructed down to the range of 500 WBC/mm^3 and overlaid on isobols of response duration or longevity, resulting in a prediction of optimum dose with greater precision perhaps than an experiment conducted in a lethal dose range.

The prediction could be further refined by repeating the procedure using platelet counts, weight loss, or other limiting toxicities. The patterns resulting from clinical studies using populations of patients would be expected to differ somewhat for the various types of toxicity. Knowledge of such patterns would allow movement away from a particular limiting toxicity in an individual patient to an equally effective but better tolerated treatment which likely would call for increasing the dose of one drug and decreasing the dose of others. This is in contrast to the current method, which usually requires the reduction of the dose of all drugs by a fixed percentage when significant toxicity occurs.

Figure 6.3 shows an example of a dual-response surface analysis. In this example, hazard contours were constructed for two experiments each for L1210 leukemia (panels A and B) and P388 leukemia (panels C and D). In a separate experiment host lethality data was obtained for the combination and a logistic model was used to construct lines representing LD_{10} and LD_{50} doses. These lines have been overlaid on each of the plots. Although the reproducibility of the contour plots is not as great as one would like, it is about what can be expected with experiments of the size employed. Each panel represents the results of 15 groups of eight animals each, plus controls.

The toxicity lines, which require fewer animals for equal reproducibility because of the simpler nature of the model employed, add materially to the interpretation of the results.

Pilot studies in humans confirm that the toxicity analyses approach statistical significance much more rapidly than the therapeutic-result analyses [14]. As multiple-toxicity parameters are always measured in clinical studies multiple-response surface analyses should become an important aspect of any response-surface experiments that may be conducted in man.

REFERENCES

1. Barranco, S. C. (1976). In vitro responses of mammalian cells to drug-induced potentially lethal and sublethal damage. *Cancer Treat. Rep., 60*, 1799-1810.

2. Barranco, S. C., and Novak, J. K. (1974). Survival responses of dividing and nondividing mammalian cells after treatment with hydroxyurea, arabinosylaytosine or adriamycin. *Cancer Res., 34*, 1616-1618.

3. Carter, W. H., Jr., Wampler, G. L., Stablein, D. M., and Campbell, E. D. (1982). Drug activity and therapeutic synergism in cancer treatment. *Cancer Res., 42*, 2963-2971.

4. DeWys, W. D. (1973). A dose-response study of resistance of leukemia L1210 to cyclophosphamide. *J. Natl. Cancer Inst., 50*, 783-789.

5. DeWys, W. D. and Knight, N. (1969). Kinetics of cyclophosphamide damage: Sublethal damage repair and cell-cycle related sensitivity. *J. Natl. Cancer Inst., 42*, 153-163.

6. Elkind, M. M. (1976). Introduction to session on drug lethality and sublethan damage: Cytotoxic damage and repair. *Cancer Treat. Rep., 60*, 1777-1780.

7. Liss, R. H., Yesair, D. W., Schepis, J. P., and Marenchic, I. C. (1977). Adriamycin and daunomycin pharmacokinetics in rats. *Proc. AACR, 18*, 221.

8. Myers, R. H. and Carter, W. H., Jr. (1973). Response surface technique for dual response systems. *Technometrics, 15*, 301-317.

9. Sabath, L. D. (1967). Synergy of antibacterial substances by apparently known mechanisms. In Antimicrobial agents and chemotherapy (G. L. Hobly, ed.), *American Society for Microbiology*, pp. 210-217.

10. Schenken, L. L. (1976). Proliferative character and growth modes of neoplastic disease as determinants of chemotherapeutic efficacy. *Cancer Treat. Rep., 60*, 1761-1776.

11. Tobey, R. A., Crissman, H. A., and Oka, M. S. (1976). Arrested and cycling CHO cells as a kinetic model: Studies with adriamycin. *Cancer Treat. Rep.*, *60*, 1829-1837.

12. Venditti, J. M. and Goldin, A. (1964). Drug synergism in antineoplastic chemotherapy. In *Advances in Chemotherapy*, Vol. 1 (A. Goldin and F. Hawkins, eds.), Academic Press, New York, pp. 397-498.

13. Venditti, J. M., Humphreys, S. R., Mantel, N., and Goldin, A. (1956). Combined treatment of advanced leukemia (L1210) in mice with amethopterin and 6-mercaptopurine. *J. Natl. Cancer Inst.*, *17*, 631-638.

14. Wampler, G. L., Carter, W. H., Jr., Glazier, R. L., and Kuperminc, M. (1979). Dose-response relationships of adriamycin (ADR) cyclophosphamide (CTX) in treatment of squamous cell carcinoma of the lung: A pilot study. *Proc. ASCO*, *20*, 401.

15. Wampler, G. L., Carter, W. H., Jr., and Williams, V. R. (1978). Combination chemotherapy: Arriving at optimal treatment levels by incorporating side effect constraints. *Cancer Treat. Rep.*, *62*, 333-340.

7

Response-Surface Exploration without Modeling

7.1 INTRODUCTION

It might appear that this text is devoted to the presentation
of statistical developments important only to the design and
analysis of preclinical combination chemotherapy experiments.
Clearly the methods discussed in the preceding chapters are
pertinent to a wider range of applications. Whenever the interest is in relating either time to response or outcome cate-
gory to continuous independent variates, the approach is
appropriate. Thus, the developments are not limited to either
animal experiments or even to the biosciences.

Unlike the previous chapters, this chapter will consider
an area of response surface exploration that requires no functional modeling of the surface to be explored. This methodology may have important implications for the evaluation of new
multi-drug combinations.

7.2 EVOLUTIONARY PROCEDURES

Of primary interest in a clinical trial is the rapid determination of the "better" treatment so that the maximum number of
patients can benefit from its use. Adaptive allocation procedures which utilize information generated during the course of
a clinical study to determine the treatment of the next patient
to enter the trial have been developed to aid in the rapid

determination of the most effective treatment. Zelen [14] has
proposed a method, "play the winner," for determining the better
of two treatments. He assumed that there are only two treatments to be compared, that patients enter the clinical trial
sequentially, and that for each patient the outcome, which depends only on the treatment, can be classified as a success or
a failure. The procedure is simple: namely, a treatment success on a given treatment is responsible for the next patient's
receiving the same treatment, while a treatment failure calls
for the next patient to receive the other treatment. Zelen
studies the properties of this simple rule and indicates that
its implementation in a clinical trial tends to place more
patients on the better treatment.

Notice that throughout this play the winner approach the
two treatments remain unchanged. For example, if the treatments
being compared are different doses of the same drug the decision
to be made is that of deciding which of the two is better--not
to gather information which might be useful in determining the
most effective dose of the drug. Similarly, if a combination
of drugs is under consideration, it is possible to determine
only which of the two combinations is better, not how to administer the drugs in the combination most effectively.

Eichorn and Zacks [8] developed a sequential-search procedure for determining the largest dose (of a single drug) for
which only a specific proportion of patients will experience
toxicity that exceeds a specific threshold. Thus, an important
difference between this procedure and play the winner is that
the former is concerned with dose determinations as opposed to
treatment comparison. Since in the determination of the next
dose level, the procedure uses information gathered on patients
already in the study, the process is an adaptive one. There
are rather strict assumptions made:

1. The relationship between dosage and toxicity is linear over a given range.
2. The conditional distribution of toxicity, given dosage levels, is Gaussian with known variance.

Eichorn and Zacks also considered a Bayesian approach to solving the problem. In a simulation study these authors showed that the estimated optimum dose in no case exceeded the optimum dose. Thus, their procedure appears to be such that the optimal treatment is approached from below, avoiding dose modifications which frequently occur in the currently used clinical-trial designs. While the approach has this desirable property, it has not been generalized to handle the more difficult problem associated with the use of a combination of drugs.

There remains the problem of designing a clinical trial to yield the optimal level of each drug in a combination. In his discussion of Mantel's [10] paper, Box [1] suggested that evolutionary operation (EVOP) may be of interest in this area. Evolutionary operation is a technique developed for use in the chemical industry as a practical way of making the transition from laboratory to production. Once in production, large changes in the production process could have a noticeable effect on the quality of the product and hence on the profitability of the operation. Therefore, any changes made in the process must be small to protect against the possibility of a noticeable decline in quality. EVOP is a procedure for searching for improved conditions while in production which proceeds through a series of small changes in conditions. If the changes have an effect, however small, with enough observations the variability in the mean response can be reduced to the point that small differences in quality become statistically significant. Once significance has been obtained, a move in the proper direction is made and the search process continues. That there is an analogy between such a process and a clinical trial is due

to ethical considerations inherent in a clinical trial. It
would not be acceptable to vary treatment widely enough to
cause toxic responses in some patients and to undertreat others
simply to view the effect of a combination treatment. Instead,
small changes in treatment levels arrived at from phase I and
phase II studies would be made, the results noted, and appropriate actions taken. In this manner the optimal way to use a
particular set of drugs in combination would evolve. Box [1]
concluded, "The method might in fact be used to get maximum
information from the normal treatment of patients by practic-
ing practitioners. It would be necessary for a central agency
to obtain agreement that doctors, in using a particular therapy
in normal practice (as contrasted with special research studies),
would vary the therapy slightly in accordance with a prescribed
plan. With a suitable statistical plan, differences arising
from small deliberate changes in the therapy can be detected
when the information is collected. In this way a steady evolu-
tion in medical practice might be set in motion to augment more
specialized research studies."

The evolutionary methods Box described were likely those
he pioneered [2]. These techniques assume an underlying normal distribution of the response variable. In many clinical
studies the response of interest is time to an event, e.g.,
time to death, length of remission, etc. Such variables are
unlikely to follow a normal distribution. Indeed, the way to
analyze such data as a function of treatment levels has been
the topic of the preceding chapters. While Box has suggested
a way of sequentially searching for the optimal treatment, the
method must be modified. Another shortcoming of the method is
the number of replications (patients) required to detect, as
significant, small changes in the response. Although EVOP offers a method for adaptively determining optimal treatment
levels, the large number of patients required necessitates

major revisions for it to be clinically useful. Perhaps the
most important feature of this approach is its ability to explore an underlying response surface without ever specifying
its functional form. In reality, with this approach we are
able to benefit from a modeling approach without making re-
strictive assumptions about the functional form of the underlying response surface.

In attempting to develop an EVOP procedure suitable for
clinical use it is necessary to mention the method of steepest
ascent. It has been found by Brooks [3] to be one of the most
efficient methods for determining the location of the optimum
of a response surface. Basically, this is a sequential procedure in which the experimenter proceeds along the path of maximum increase in response. The steps to the procedure can be
described as follows:

1. The researcher approximates the underlying response
    surface for the experimental data by a first-degree
    polynomial in a restricted region of the treatment
    space.

2. From the information obtained in Step 1, the path of
    steepest ascent is estimated and a new experiment is
    performed in a region some fixed distance from the
    preceding experimental region along the path of
    steepest ascent.

3. Steps 1 and 2 are repeated until no further gain in
    response can be obtained.

This process is presented graphically in Fig. 7.1.

Of particular interest in the method is the size of the
experiment, i.e., the number of observations in each of the
sequentially determined experimental regions. It would appear
that the process would benefit from the precise estimates of
the direction of steepest ascent which would result from larger
experiments in each region. Brooks and Mickey [4] showed, surprisingly, that for a normally distributed response variable
and a planar response function that the optimal number of

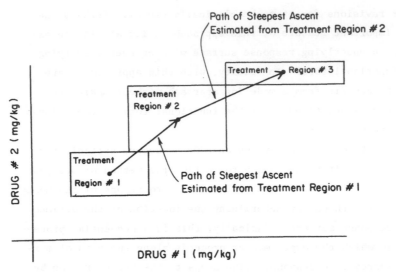

FIGURE 7.1. Graphic representation of the method of steepest ascent.

trials in any region along the path of steepest ascent is equal
to one more than the number of independent variables. In other
words, it is not worthwhile to replicate the experiment to effect an increase in the precision of the estimate of the direction of steepest ascent at the expense of additional experiments
along the path of steepest ascent. This result was obtained
independently of the magnitude of the variability of the underlying response. Although clinical trial data are not generally
normally distributed about a planar model, the result is encour-
aging in that it suggests a way to reduce the number of patients
required to determine via a clinical trial the optimum doses of
each drug in a combination.

Spendley, Hext, and Himsworth [13] proposed simplex EVOP
as an automatic procedure which would attain the optimality
conditions in a k-dimensional process more rapidly than the
EVOP procedure developed by Box. The use of this technique in

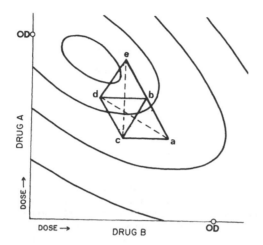

FIGURE 7.2. Graphic representation of simplex EVOP.

the determination of the dosages of two drugs associated with maximum response is illustrated in Fig. 7.2.

The procedure begins by comparing the responses observed at three different combinations a, b, and c of two drugs. In the figure the response at combination a is seen to be the smallest of the three. As a result a new point, d, is determined as the reflection of a through the midpoint of the line segment connecting b and c. In this manner progress toward the optimum combination is made by moving away from the minimum response. (It can be shown that the procedure is a primitive form of the steepest ascent method discussed earlier.) By comparing the response at b, c, and d it can be determined that the response at point c is the minimum. As a result, the method calls for a reflection away from c through the line joining b and d to point e. This process continues until further improvement in response cannot be detected.

This procedure is easily generalized to permit the optimization of a k-variable process by permitting reflections away

from the smallest response observed at the k + 1 vertices of a
k-dimensional simplex. (In two dimensions a triangle is a simplex; in three dimensions, a tetrahedron.) There are several
advantages associated with the use of this procedure:

1. Since the direction of advance is dependent only on
   the ranking of the observations, the procedure can be
   used with qualitative and quantitative response
   variables.

2. The procedure can be used to obtain optimum responses
   in the presence of constraints.

3. Carpenter and Sweeny [6] found that this procedure
   made the most progress per observational unit when no
   replication occurred, as long as the ratio of the gradient of the underlying response surface to the standard deviation was greater than 0.5. Thus, it does not
   require a large number of observations at each point
   in the treatment space before a change is made.

Segreti [1] and Segreti, Carter, and Wampler [12] considered use of the method of steepest ascent and simplex EVOP in
the development of adaptive methods for estimating the optimal
levels of each component in a combination of cytotoxic agents.
These authors considered procedures specifically for the clinical situation in which a group of agents has shown activity for
a particular tumor and in which the best combination of these
drugs is unknown. As a result of properties of these drugs determined, for example, in phase I and phase II studies, a treatment region is chosen. Combinations located in this region are
selected for the initial experimental design. As patients enter
the study they are randomly assigned to these treatment combinations. After a predetermined period of follow-up the data are
analyzed. Guided by the results of such analysis the experimental region is moved in the direction of improved response. The
sequence of patient accrual, data analysis, and determination
of new regions of experimentation is continued indefinitely.
With such a procedure it is possible, as a result of random
fluctuation, to move to a region of inferior response. However,

it should be noted that the procedure as described is self-correcting in that the next step is likely to be associated with a return to a region of improved response. As long as the step size used to move from one region to the other, i.e., the difference in dosage levels from one region to the next, is not too large, there is no ethical consequence of such a misguided step, since whenever movement occurs there is an indication that it is in the direction of improved response. By restricting the step size the risk of stepping past the optimal combination is reduced. Thus, the procedure is essentially an evolutionary one without the testing of hypotheses associated with Box's approach.

In each of the procedures considered by Segreti [11] and Segreti, Carter, and Wampler [12], the response of interest was taken to be the mean failure rate per fixed time period

$$\hat{\lambda}_j = \frac{\sum_{i=1}^{m_j} d_{ij}}{\sum_{i=1}^{m_j} t_{ij}}$$

where

$\hat{\lambda}_j$ = the estimated mean failure rate for jth treatment combination

d_{ij} = an indicator variable which takes on a value of 1 if the ith individual in the jth treatment group fails and 0 otherwise

t_{ij} = time the ith person in the jth group is on study

m_j = number of individuals randomized to the jth treatment group

Since most studies involving time to response data include some censored observations as well as complete data, it is important that censored observations be included in the computation of $\hat{\lambda}_j$. For example, consider the following set of failure times:

1, 2, 3^+, 4, 4^+, 5, 5^+, where the censored observations are denoted by a + superscript. With these data:

$$\hat{\lambda} = \frac{4}{1 + 2 + 3 + 4 + 4 + 5 + 5}$$

$$= \frac{4}{24}$$

$$= 0.167$$

If the data come from an underlying exponential distribution $\hat{\lambda}_j$ is the maximum-likelihood estimate of the hazard rate of the jth treatment group. Otherwise, Cutler and Myers [7] point out that this statistic can be interpreted as the average mortality rate for the jth group over the observational period. Thus, as a result of the adaptive methods, there should be movement in the direction of dosage levels associated with lower mean failure rates.

The initial method, called SAND (steepest ascent, new data), is based on the direct use of the method of steepest ascent. Here the underlying response surface, in a narrow region of the treatment space, is approximated by a first-degree polynomial in order that the direction of steepest ascent can be estimated. From this, a new region in the treatment space along this path is determined. Subjects are randomly assigned treatment in the new region, and after a fixed period of time only the data from the latest region are analyzed. The direction of steepest ascent is estimated and the site of yet another experimental region is located. In the situation for which these techniques are designed the available information is limited. Generally, the small number of available patients, the variability in the time to response due to various uncontrolled and unknown factors, and censoring all combine to complicate the process of estimating optimal levels of treatment. Thus, SAND's use of only the most current data in estimating the direction of steepest ascent is rather extravagant. As a result, a different procedure, SAPD (steepest ascent, previous data), was considered. Here information from the previous four experiments is used in estimating the path of steepest ascent. It should be noted that SAPD, as a result of the use of this previous data, depends more strongly than SAND on the assumption that the underlying response surface can be approximated by a first-degree polynomial. But in the situation where this assumption is valid SAPD should be more reliable than SAND as a result of the more efficient use of the available information. The inclusion of the earlier patients will result in the use of more complete information, in that these data are less likely to be censored since they have been on study for a greater period of time. The third method considered (SIMP) is a modification of the simplex EVOP procedure developed by Spendley, Hext, and Himsworth [13]. Here patients are randomized to one of $k + 1$ different combinations of the k drugs. After a predetermined time the group with largest $\hat{\lambda}$ is determined. Since $\hat{\lambda}_j$ can be computed in the presence of censored observations accrual can occur continuously. This is in contrast to the play the winner process, the use of which can be complicated by the appearance of a new case before a winner has been determined. A new treatment combination is determined by reflecting away from this point. An exception occurs if reflection would result in the replication of the immediately preceding rejected point. In this case reflection is made from the combination with second largest $\hat{\lambda}$. Spendley, Hext, and Himsworth also recommend the replication of any point which has occurred in $k + 1$ previous sets of treatment combinations, since such a treatment could appear to be superior as a result of random events. If such is the case, replication is likely to suggest movement from that point. However, in the clinical trial application the accrual and assignment process allows for the continual remeasurement of the response variable, e.g., a censored observation at one

stage of the process likely will not remain so throughout the
study, and hence such a procedure is not as necessary.

Segreti, Carter, and Wampler [12] compared the performance
of these three methods in a Monte Carlo study. They simulated
a clinical trial in which the expected number of patient accruals was two per week. Following a suggestion by George and
Désu [9] that patient accruals in a clinical trial follow a
Poisson process, the actual number of entries per week was distributed as a Poisson random variable with a mean of two
patients per week. Patients were allowed to enter for 26 weeks.
After this period the data were analyzed, the experimental region was changed as the analysis indicated, and accrual continued. As described, this process simulates a trial which admits
approximately 100 patients per year. Analysis occurs after six
months of accrual and every six months thereafter. The progress
made toward the optimal combination was measured at the end of
two years (i.e., after four 26-week time intervals had elapsed),
five years, and ten years. For the purposes of the simulation
an observation was censored if the time to response after entry
was greater than the time point at which the analysis was to
occur. As they occurred the observations were randomized among
the $k + 1$ treatment groups required to study a combination of k
drugs for both SAND and SAPD. Recall that the simplex search
procedure (SIMP) requires addition of a single point to K points
from the previous design to form the new treatment space. To
balance the available information, the simulations were designed
so that the observations were assigned to the new treatment
point with a probability of 0.5 and each of the k remaining
points was assigned with a probability of $0.5/k$.

The simulation study compared the three procedures in two
different situations. Since each of the procedures, to varying
degrees, assumes a locally planar response surface, it was decided to determine first how they performed when the underlying

relationship between the failure rate and dosage levels in a
two-drug combination was linear and the underlying distribution
was exponential. Since the fitted response surface and the
underlying surface are of the same form and since the measured
response the failure rate $\hat{\lambda}$ can be justified from an exponential distribution, it should be expected that the methods would
perform rather well. The comparison was facilitated by calcu-
lating for each of the methods the maximum gain after various
lengths of time. The gain was defined as the change in the
mean survival times of the treatments, which had evolved after
various time intervals for which the method had been in use.
The results were

    SAPD > SIMP > SAND

after allowing the procedures to operate for time periods equivalent to two years, five years, and ten years. This ordering
was independent of the amount of censoring associated with the
data.

It is not surprising that under these circumstances SAPD
performs better than either SIMP or SAND. This follows since
SAPD assumes a planar surface over a larger region of treatment
space than does either of the two other procedures. Somewhat
surprisingly, SIMP performed better than SAND. Finally, it
could be seen that SIMP and SAPD were not affected by censoring
to the same degree as was SAND. The authors speculate that
this is because the first two procedures retain information
from one region to another while SAND discards information at
each move from one region to another. When the number of drugs
considered in combination increased from two to four there was
no change in the results.

After studying the performance of these techniques on data
resulting from an exponential distribution whose parameter was
a first-degree polynomial in the dosage levels, the authors

considered the same methods on data from an exponential distribution whose parameter was quadratic in the dosage levels of
the two drugs. Interestingly, the same ordering among the
three procedures was observed as in the linear case. Although
SAPD assumes an underlying first-degree relationship between
dosage levels and response when in fact a second-degree relationship is in effect, it appears that the more complete use
of the experimental data counteracts the effect of the model
misspecification. When the number of independent variables in
the quadratic relationship, i.e., the number of drugs in the
combinations, was increased from two to four there was no
change in the results.

It appears that SAPD and SIMP can be used effectively to
produce improved treatments when the exponential distribution
describes the survival patterns of treated patients. However,
since the response used, the average failure rate, is the maximum-likelihood estimator of the parameter of the underlying
exponential distribution, it could be argued that if the methods worked at all they should work under these conditions. It
is, therefore, important to study the performance of these
methods when the underlying distribution is other than
exponential.

Segreti, Carter, and Wampler [12] considered the robust-
ness of these methods to variations in the underlying distribution in a simulation study. These authors used the Weibull
distribution with increasing and decreasing hazard functions.
As in their earlier study, the simulation was designed to re-
semble a clinical trial which enters an average of two patients
per week with provisions for analyses every six months. The
relationship between survival and treatment levels was developed through Cox's proportional hazard model [5] by considering
a relative hazard function which is quadratic in the dosage
levels. This is a reasonable approximation to reality, in that

as treatment levels increase from zero through the therapeutic range to toxic levels, it is likely that the hazard will decrease until a minimum is reached and then increase. Thus, for a two-drug combination the assumed hazard function takes the form $\lambda(t) = \lambda_0(t)\psi(x_1, x_2)$, where $\lambda_0(t)$ is the hazard function of the Weibull distribution and $\psi(x_1, x_2)$ is a quadratic function of the doses of drugs 1 and 2 of the form $\beta_1 x_1^2 + \beta_2 x_2^2$, with values of β_1 and β_2 specified.

The efficiency of the three methods was measured by the percentage of possible improvement in the relative hazard function. Let ψ_i be the relative hazard at the center of the initial simplex and ψ_0 be the optimum (minimum) value of the same function. Then, if after k six-month time intervals the procedure in question has led to a treatment with a relative hazard of ψ_k, the percent of possible gain is

$$100 \, \frac{\psi_k - \psi_i}{\psi_0 - \psi_i}$$

For the increasing hazard function in the simulation study, SAPD had a higher percentage of possible gain than SIMP, which performed better than SAND; after both four and ten cycles (i.e., after two to five years) both SIMP and SAND continued to find more effective treatments while SAPD was unable to maintain the progress it had made earlier. When the decreasing failure rate was used in the simulations SAPD and SAND resulted in substantial progress with SAND making slightly less progress than SAPD. Of the three procedures SIMP performed poorest in this situation.

Although at the present time clinical trials are not used to optimize treatment levels it does appear that adaptive or evolutionary techniques can be modified in such a way that can be of clinical use. Indeed, these types of trial may have unique advantages. Ethically they are such that every patient receives either a treatment that is acceptable according to present standards or one for which there is an indication of superiority to the currently accepted treatment. Importantly, they promote the systematic exploration of the underlying treatment-response surface. This exploration would appear to lead to a better understanding of how the treatment agents interact with each other and how they jointly affect the disease.

REFERENCES

1. Box, G. E. P. (1958). In Discussion of experimental design in combination chemotherapy. *Ann. N.Y. Acad. Sci.*, *76*, 909-931.

2. Box, G. E. P. (1957). Evolutionary operation: A method for increasing industrial productivity. *App. Stat.*, *6*, 81-101.

3. Brooks, S. H. (1959). A comparison of maximum seeking methods. *Operations Res.*, *7*, 430-457.

4. Brooks, S. H., and Mickey, M. R. (1961). Optimum estimation of gradient direction in steepest ascent experiments. *Biometrics*, *17*, 48-56.

5. Cox, D. R. (1972). Regression models and life tables. *J. Roy. Stat. Soc. B*, *34*, 187-220.

6. Carpenter, B. C. and Sweeny, H. C. (1965). Process improvement with "simplex" self directing evolutionary operation. *Chem. Eng.*, *72*, 117-126.

7. Cutler, S. J. and Myers, M. H. (1967). Clinical classification of extent of disease in cancer of the breast. *J. Nat. Cancer Inst.*, *39*, 193-207.

8. Eichorn, B. H. and Zacks, S. (1973). Sequential search of an optimal dosage, I. *J. Amer. Stat. Assoc.*, *68*, 594-598.

9. George, S. L. and Desu, M. M. (1973). Planning the size and duration of a trial studying the time to some critical event. *J. Chronic Diseases*, *27*, 15-24.

10. Mantel, N. (1958). Experimental design in combination chemotherapy. *Ann. N.Y. Acad. Sci.*, *76*, 909-931.

11. Segreti, A. C. (1977). The design of sequential clinical trials in combination chemotherapy. Unpublished doctoral dissertation, Medical College of Virginia, Virginia Commonwealth University, Richmond.

12. Segreti, A. C., Carter, W. H., and Wampler, G. L. (1979).
     Monte Carlo evaluation of several sequential optimization
     techniques when the response is time to an event. *J.
     Stat. Comp. and Simul.*, *9*, 289-301.

13. Spendley, W., Hext, G. R., and Himsworth, F. R. (1962).
     Sequential application of simplex designs in optimization
     and EVOP. *Technometrics*, *4*, 441-461.

14. Zelen, M. (1969). Play-the-winner rule and the controlled
     clinical trial. *J. Amer. Stat. Assoc.*, *64*, 131-146.

Appendix

LISTING AND EXAMPLES OF COMPUTER PROGRAMS

To illustrate application of the methodology presented in Chaps.
2 and 3, data from a two-drug combination were analyzed using
both the logistic regression model and the proportional hazards
model. Following are listings of computer programs and sub-
routines used and output subsequently obtained. Comments are
included to facilitate understanding but are not necessary for
the use of the programs. The experimental data are contained
in Table A.1.

TABLE A.1. Survival and Treatment Data from 5-FU/ CTX Experiment (148)

TREATMENT(MG/KG)		SURVIVAL TIMES
5FU	CTX	DAYS
0	0	10(2),11(5),12
100	0	13,14(2),15(2)
150	0	14(3),15(4),17
225	0	13,14,15(5),16
338	0	16(3),17(3),18(2)
500	0	13(2),16,17(4),18
0	100	10,20(4),21,22,27
0	150	20(3),21(2),23(3)
0	225	20,21(2),22(2),29,31,34
0	338	10,20,21(2),23,32,37,41
0	500	14,18,30,34,92,103,117
100	100	17,20(3),22,36,117+(2)
100	150	9,13,23(4),26(2)
100	225	20,24,26,27(2),28,30,33
100	338	14(2),21,23,26,35,37,46
150	100	17,20,21(2),23(2),25,27
150	150	23(2),25(2),26(2),28,30
150	225	16,20(2),23,28,30,34,37
150	338	13,15,22,28,34,41,43
225	100	18,20(2),21(2),22,23(2)
225	150	22,23(2),26,41,117+(3)
225	225	10,14,17(2),20,27,30
225	338	13(2),14,15,18,30,37,41
338	100	14,15,16,17,20,22,23(2)
338	150	14,15,16,17,18(4)
338	225	14,15(3),17,18,20
338	338	12(2),13,14(4),17

The number in parentheses indicates the number of deaths on that day.

LOGISTIC REGRESSION ANALYSIS

This is a SAS (Statistical Analysis System) program written to analyze a two-drug combination experiment. For additional information concerning SAS the reader is referred to [2]. To perform the logistic regression, the LOGIST procedure is utilized. Additionally, the program calculates the χ^2 goodness-of-fit test, plots contours of constant response for the two drugs and plots the estimated confidence region for the optimal combination of the two drugs. Definitions for the eight "MACRO"s, explained on comment cards at the beginning of the program, must be supplied by the user. Data is read from cards which should follow the "CARDS" statement. Cards should be punched in the following manner, each value separated from the next by at least one blank. The example cards to follow are taken from the data in Table A.1. Each line represents one card, which contains all the input information for one subject: group number, survival time, dose of first drug, dose of second drug.

1	10	0	0
1	10	0	0
1	11	0	0
1	11	0	0
1	11	0	0
1	11	0	0
1	11	0	0
1	12	0	0
2	13	100	0
2	14	100	0
2	14	100	0
.	.	.	.
.	.	.	.
.	.	.	.
27	12	338	338
27	12	338	338
27	13	338	338
27	14	338	338
27	14	338	338
27	14	338	338
27	14	338	338
27	17	338	338

For this experiment, having 209 subjects apportioned to 27
groups with two treatments, CPU time used on an IBM-168,
running MVS, was approximately one minute.

```
// EXEC SAS,REGION=1024K
//SAS.SYSIN DD *
*********************************************************************************!
*                                                                               !
*     LOGISTIC REGRESSION ANALYSIS, GOODNESS-OF-FIT TEST AND DENSITY PLOT        !
*                                                                               !
*********************************************************************************!
*                                                                               !
OPTIONS LEAVE=10000;
*                                                                               !
*THE FOLLOWING MACRO DEFINITIONS ARE SET BY THE USER FOR EACH RUN:              !
*   NAMETITL    TITLE IDENTIFYING EXPERIMENT ANALYZED IN THIS RUN               !
*   FAVOUTCM    DAY ON OR BEYOND WHICH SURVIVAL IS CONSIDERED A FAVORABLE OUTCOME!
*               (E.G., TWICE THE MEDIAN SURVIVAL TIME FOR CONTROL GROUP)         !
*   TERMS       LIST OF INDEPENDENT VARIABLES IN THE MODEL                       !
*   NUMPARAM    NUMBER OF PARAMETERS IN THE MODEL INCLUDING INTERCEPT PARAMETER  !
*   DRUG1       NAME OF VARIABLE 'X1' WHICH IS THE FIRST DRUG IN THE COMBINATION !
*   DRUG2       NAME OF VARIABLE 'X2' WHICH IS THE SECOND DRUG IN THE COMBINATION!
*   HORIZMAX    A NUMBER <= HIGHEST DOSAGE LEVEL OF DRUG1,  USED TO DEFINE RANGE !
*               OF HORIZONTAL AXIS FOR PLOT                                      !
*   VERTMAX     A NUMBER <= HIGHEST DOSAGE LEVEL OF DRUG2,  USED TO DEFINE RANGE !
*               OF VERTICAL AXIS FOR PLOT                                        !
*                                                                               !
*                                                                               !
MACRO NAMETITL EXPERIMENT 148 - 5FU, CTX%
MACRO FAVOUTCM 22.0%
MACRO TERMS X1 X2 X1SQ X2SQ X1X2%
MACRO NUMPARAM 6%
MACRO DRUG1 _5FU%
MACRO DRUG2 CTX%
MACRO HORIZMAX 500%
MACRO VERTMAX 500%
*                                                                               !
*-------------------------------------------------------------------------------!
*                                                                               !
*     LOGISTIC REGRESSION ANALYSIS                                              !
*                                                                               !
*-------------------------------------------------------------------------------!
*                                                                               !
TITLE LOGISTIC REGRESSION ANALYSIS OF NAMETITL;
*                                                                               !
*READ DATA IN FOLLOWING STEP:                                                   !
*   GROUP       TREATMENT GROUP TO WHICH SUBJECT BELONGS                        !
*   SURVTIME    TIME TO FAILURE                                                 !
*   X1          DOSE OF FIRST DRUG IN THE COMBINATION                           !
*   X2          DOSE OF SECOND DRUG IN THE COMBINATION                          !
*                                                                               !
DATA ORIGINAL;
  INPUT GROUP SURVTIME X1 X2;
*                                                                               !
*DETERMINE DEPENDENT VARIABLE 'RESPONSE',  '1' INDICATES A FAVORABLE OUTCOME,   !
*               '0' INDICATES AN UNFAVORABLE OUTCOME.                           !
*                                                                               !
  IF SURVTIME < FAVOUTCM THEN RESPONSE=0;
  IF SURVTIME >= FAVOUTCM THEN RESPONSE=1;
*                                                                               !
*CALCULATE VALUES OF REMAINING INDEPENDENT VARIABLES IN MODEL                   !
*                                                                               !
  X1SQ = X1*X1;
  X2SQ = X2*X2;
```

```
    X1X2 = X1*X2;
    LABEL RESPONSE=SURVIVAL LONGER THAN FAVOUTCM DAYS;
    CARDS;
*
*DATA CARDS GO HERE                                                             ;
*                                                                               ;
*'PROC MEANS' USED TO CALCULATE AND OUTPUT TO DATASET MINIMUM VALUES AND         ;
*               RANGES OF DOSAGE LEVELS OF DRUGS                                 ;
*                                                                               ;
*                                                                               ;
PROC MEANS NOPRINT; VAR X1 X2;                                                   ;
    OUTPUT OUT=DIMENS MIN=MIN_X1 MIN_X2 RANGE=RANGE_X1 RANGE_X2;
*
*'PROC LOGIST' USED TO PERFORM ANALYSIS, TO OUTPUT ESTIMATES AND COVARIANCE      ;
*               MATRIX TO DATASET 'BETAS' AND TO OUTPUT PREDICTED PROBABILITY    ;
*               OF FAVORABLE OUTCOME (ALONG WITH ITS 95% CONFIDENCE LIMITS) FOR  ;
*               EACH OBSERVATION TO DATASET 'PRED'                              ;
*MODEL DEFINED IN MACRO 'TERMS' AT BEGINNING OF PROGRAM                          ;
*
PROC LOGIST DATA=ORIGINAL OUTPUT OUT=BETAS OUTPUTP OUTP=PRED(RENAME=(_P_=PROB))  ;
    PRINTC;
    MODEL RESPONSE = TERMS;
*
*-----------------------------------------------------------------------------; ;
*                                                                               ;
*     CALCULATION OF CHI-SQUARED GOODNESS-OF-FIT TEST                            ;
*                                                                               ;
*-----------------------------------------------------------------------------; ;
*                                                                               ;
DATA GOODFIT;
    SET PRED;
    PQ = PROB*(1-PROB);
    ANIMAL = _N_;
PROC SORT; BY GROUP;
PROC PRINT; VAR GROUP X1 X2 SURVTIME RESPONSE _LOWER_ PROB _UPPER_;
    ID ANIMAL;
    TITLE3 ''PROB'' IS PREDICTED PROBABILITY OF SURVIVAL LONGER THAN FAVOUTCM DAYS
    ;
*
*'PROC MEANS' USED TO CALCULATE OBERVED AND EXPECTED FREQUENCIES OF              ;
*               FAVORABLE OUTCOMES FOR EACH TREATMENT GROUP AND DENOMINATOR OF   ;
*               GROUP CHI-SQUARE                                                 ;
*                                                                               ;
PROC MEANS NOPRINT SUM; BY GROUP X1 X2;
    VAR PROB RESPONSE PQ;
    OUTPUT OUT=SUMS SUM=EXPECTED OBSERVED SUMPQ;
*
*CALCULATING GROUP CHI-SQUARES                                                   ;
*                                                                               ;
DATA CHI2;
    SET SUMS;
    NUM = (EXPECTED - OBSERVED)**2;
    GRPCHI = NUM/SUMPQ;
PROC PRINT; VAR X1 X2 EXPECTED OBSERVED GRPCHI; ID GROUP;
    TITLE3 ;
    TITLE7 GOODNESS-OF-FIT STATISTICS;
PROC MEANS NOPRINT; VAR GRPCHI; OUTPUT OUT=FINAL N=NUMGRPS SUM=CHISQ;
*
*CALCULATING AND PRINTING OVERALL CHI-SQUARE TEST STATISTIC, DEGREES OF          ;
*               FREEDOM, P-VALUES AND NUMBER OF GROUPS                           ;
```

```
*
DATA CHISQTST;
  SET FINAL;
  DF = NUMGRPS - NUMPARAM;
  P = 1 - PROBCHI(CHISQ,DF);
  FILE PRINT;
  PUT //// @ 20 CHISQ= P= DF= NUMGRPS=;
*                                                                              |
*------------------------------------------------------------------------------|
*                                                                              |
*     PLOT OF CONTOURS OF CONSTANT RESPONSE FOR COMBINATION OF TWO DRUGS        |
*                                                                              |
*------------------------------------------------------------------------------|
*                                                                              |
DATA BETANEW;
  MERGE BETAS DIMENS;
*                                                                              |
*DATA STEP 'PLOTIT' AND MACRO 'PROCESS' GENERATE THE GRID OF OBSERVATIONS FOR   |
*                THE PLOT AND CALCULATE THE ESTIMATED PROBABILITY OF A FAVORABLE |
*                OUTCOME AT EACH POINT                                          |
*                                                                              |
MACRO PROCESS
  X = MIN_X1 + IO * RANGE_X1;
  Y = MIN_X2 + JO * RANGE_X2;
  XPB= INTERCEP + X1*X + X2*Y + X1SQ*(X**2) + X2SQ*(Y**2) + X1X2*X*Y;
  P = 1 / (1 + EXP(-XPB));
  FORMAT P 5.3;
  OUTPUT;
%
DATA PLOTIT;
  SET BETANEW;
  IF _N_=1;
  X=MIN_X1; Y=MIN_X2; P=0.0; OUTPUT;
  X=0.0; Y=0.0; P=1.0; OUTPUT;
  DO I = 0 TO 100;
    IO = I/100;
    DO J = 0 TO 50;
      JO = J/50;
      PROCESS;
      END;
    END;
DATA REDUCED;
  SET PLOTIT;
  IF X<=HORIZMAX AND Y<=VERTMAX;
  RENAME X=DRUG1 Y=DRUG2;
PROC PLOT;
  PLOT DRUG2*DRUG1=P / CONTOUR=10;
  TITLE3  ;
*                                                                              |
*------------------------------------------------------------------------------|
*                                                                              |
*     PLOT OF ESTIMATED CONFIDENCE REGION FOR THE OPTIMUM COMBINATION OF        |
*                TWO DRUGS                                                      |
*                                                                              |
*------------------------------------------------------------------------------|
*                                                                              |
PROC MATRIX;
FETCH BIGMAT DATA=BETANEW;
NR=NROW(BIGMAT);
NC = NCOL(BIGMAT);
```

```
NC = NC - 4;
NEWMAT = BIGMAT(1:NR,2:NC);
XC = NC - 1;
B = NEWMAT(1,1:XC);
V = NEWMAT(3:NR,1:XC);
MIN_X1 = BIGMAT(1,7);
MIN_X2 = BIGMAT(1,8);
RANGE_X1 = BIGMAT(1,9);
RANGE_X2 = BIGMAT(1,10);
MAX_X1 = MIN_X1 + RANGE_X1;
MAX_X2 = MIN_X2 + RANGE_X2;
ZZ = MIN_X1//MIN_X2//0;
ZZ = ZZ';
DO X1 = MIN_X1 TO MAX_X1 BY RANGE_X1 #/50;
  DO X2 = MIN_X2 TO MAX_X2 BY RANGE_X2 #/50;
    L1   = B(1,1) + 2*B(1,3)*X1 + B(1,5)*X2;
    L2   = B(1,2) + 2*B(1,4)*X2 + B(1,5)*X1;
    VAR1 = V(1,1) + 4*(X1**2)*V(3,3) + (X2**2)*V(5,5) + 4*X1*V(1,3)
         + 2*X2*V(1,5) + 4*X1*X2*V(3,5);
    VAR2 = V(2,2) + 4*(X2**2)*V(4,4) + (X1**2)*V(5,5) + 4*X2*V(2,4)
         + 2*X1*V(2,5) + 4*X1*X2*V(4,5);
    VAR12 = V(1,2) + 2*X2*V(1,4) + X1*V(1,5) + 2*X1*V(2,3) + 4*X1*X2*V(3,4)
         + 2*(X1**2)*V(3,5) + X2*V(2,5) + 2*(X2**2)*V(4,5) + X1*X2*V(5,5);
    L = L1//L2;
    VA = VAR1//VAR12;
    VB = VAR12//VAR2;
    VCVL = VA'//VB';
    Y = L'*INV(VCVL)*L;
    W = 0;  IF Y<5.99 THEN W=1;
    Z = X1//X2//W;
    ZZ = ZZ//Z';
  END;
END;
OUTPUT ZZ OUT=NEW (RENAME=(COL1=DRUG1 COL2=DRUG2));
PROC PLOT;
PLOT DRUG2*DRUG1=COL3 / CONTOUR=2;
TITLE3 ESTIMATED CONFIDENCE REGION;
//
```

The following is the computer output from the preceding program, using the data given in Table A.1.

LOGISTIC REGRESSION ANALYSIS OF EXPERIMENT 148 - 5FU, CTX

LOGISTIC REGRESSION PROCEDURE

DEPENDENT VARIABLE: RESPONSE   SURVIVAL LONGER THAN 22.0 DAYS

```
        209 OBSERVATIONS
         82 POSITIVES
        127 NEGATIVES
          0 OBSERVATIONS DELETED DUE TO MISSING VALUES
```

VARIABLE	MEAN	MINIMUM	MAXIMUM	RANGE
X1	169.89	0	500	500
X2	168.574	0	500	500
X1SQ	46303.3	0	250000	250000
X2SQ	45116.1	0	250000	250000
X1X2	24451.6	0	114244	114244

-2 LOG LIKELIHOOD FOR MODEL CONTAINING INTERCEPT ONLY= 279.97

```
CONVERGENCE OBTAINED IN  6 ITERATIONS,                D=0.293,
MAX ABSOLUTE DERIVATIVE=0.1262D+02,        -2 LOG L= 196.03,
MODEL CHI-SQUARE=   83.94 WITH   5 D.F.           P=0.0   .
```

VARIABLE	BETA	STD. ERROR	CHI-SQUARE	P	D
INTERCEPT	-5.18048786	1.13824898	20.71	0.0000	
X1	0.03163901	0.00784159	16.28	0.0001	0.074
X2	0.03880772	0.00814548	22.70	0.0000	0.101
X1SQ	-0.00007277	0.00001708	18.16	0.0000	0.082
X2SQ	-0.00005707	0.00001314	18.85	0.0000	0.085
X1X2	-0.00007392	0.00002172	11.58	0.0007	0.054

CLASSIFICATION TABLE

PREDICTED

		NEGATIVE	POSITIVE	TOTAL
TRUE	NEGATIVE	100	27	127
	POSITIVE	23	59	82
	TOTAL	123	86	209

```
SENSITIVITY: 72.0%  SPECIFICITY: 78.7%  CORRECT: 76.1%
FALSE POSITIVE RATE: 31.4%  FALSE NEGATIVE RATE: 18.7%
PREDICTIVE ACCURACY COEFFICIENT: 0.323
```

LOGISTIC REGRESSION ANALYSIS OF EXPERIMENT 148 - 5FU, CTX

LOGISTIC REGRESSION PROCEDURE

DEPENDENT VARIABLE: RESPONSE SURVIVAL LONGER THAN 22.0 DAYS

COVARIANCE MATRIX OF ESTIMATES

	INTERCEP	X1	X2	X1SQ	X2SQ	X1X2
INTERCEP	1.295611	-0.00714445	-0.00836761	.00000919069	.00001168011	.00002063233
X1	-0.00714445	.00006149058	.00003785562	-1.14203E-07	-4.66423E-08	-1.29496E-07
X2	-0.00836761	.00003785562	.00006634884	-3.72409E-08	-1.02686E-07	-1.44650E-07
X1SQ	.00000919069	-1.14203E-07	-3.72409E-08	2.91630E-10	3.93488E-11	1.44571E-10
X2SQ	.00001168011	-4.66423E-08	-1.02686E-07	3.93488E-11	1.72722E-10	1.98800E-10
X1X2	.00002063233	-1.29496E-07	-1.44650E-07	1.44571E-10	1.98800E-10	4.71650E-10

LOGISTIC REGRESSION ANALYSIS OF EXPERIMENT 148 = 5FU, CTX

'PROB' IS PREDICTED PROBABILITY OF SURVIVAL LONGER THAN 22.0 DAYS

ANIMAL	GROUP	X1	X2	SURVTIME	RESPONSE	_LOWER_	PROB	_UPPER_
1	1	0	0	10	0	0.0006	0.0056	0.0498
2	1	0	0	10	0	0.0006	0.0056	0.0498
3	1	0	0	11	0	0.0006	0.0056	0.0498
4	1	0	0	11	0	0.0006	0.0056	0.0498
5	1	0	0	11	0	0.0006	0.0056	0.0498
6	1	0	0	11	0	0.0006	0.0056	0.0498
7	1	0	0	11	0	0.0006	0.0056	0.0498
8	1	0	0	12	0	0.0006	0.0056	0.0498
9	2	100	0	13	0	0.0166	0.0604	0.1969
10	2	100	0	14	0	0.0166	0.0604	0.1969
11	2	100	0	14	0	0.0166	0.0604	0.1969
12	2	100	0	15	0	0.0166	0.0604	0.1969
13	2	100	0	15	0	0.0166	0.0604	0.1969
14	3	150	0	14	0	0.0395	0.1118	0.2784
15	3	150	0	14	0	0.0395	0.1118	0.2784
16	3	150	0	14	0	0.0395	0.1118	0.2784
17	3	150	0	15	0	0.0395	0.1118	0.2784
18	3	150	0	15	0	0.0395	0.1118	0.2784
19	3	150	0	15	0	0.0395	0.1118	0.2784
20	3	150	0	15	0	0.0395	0.1118	0.2784
21	3	150	0	17	0	0.0395	0.1118	0.2784
22	4	225	0	13	0	0.0593	0.1486	0.3257
23	4	225	0	14	0	0.0593	0.1486	0.3257
24	4	225	0	15	0	0.0593	0.1486	0.3257
25	4	225	0	15	0	0.0593	0.1486	0.3257
26	4	225	0	15	0	0.0593	0.1486	0.3257
27	4	225	0	15	0	0.0593	0.1486	0.3257
28	4	225	0	15	0	0.0593	0.1486	0.3257
29	4	225	0	16	0	0.0593	0.1486	0.3257
30	5	338	0	16	0	0.0135	0.0573	0.2123
31	5	338	0	16	0	0.0135	0.0573	0.2123
32	5	338	0	16	0	0.0135	0.0573	0.2123
33	5	338	0	17	0	0.0135	0.0573	0.2123
34	5	338	0	17	0	0.0135	0.0573	0.2123
35	5	338	0	17	0	0.0135	0.0573	0.2123
36	5	338	0	18	0	0.0135	0.0573	0.2123
37	5	338	0	18	0	0.0135	0.0573	0.2123
38	6	500	0	13	0	0.0000	0.0005	0.0233
39	6	500	0	13	0	0.0000	0.0005	0.0233
40	6	500	0	16	0	0.0000	0.0005	0.0233
41	6	500	0	17	0	0.0000	0.0005	0.0233
42	6	500	0	17	0	0.0000	0.0005	0.0233
43	6	500	0	17	0	0.0000	0.0005	0.0233
44	6	500	0	17	0	0.0000	0.0005	0.0233
45	6	500	0	18	0	0.0000	0.0005	0.0233
46	7	0	100	10	0	0.0475	0.1335	0.3225
47	7	0	100	20	0	0.0475	0.1335	0.3225
48	7	0	100	20	0	0.0475	0.1335	0.3225
49	7	0	100	20	0	0.0475	0.1335	0.3225
50	7	0	100	20	0	0.0475	0.1335	0.3225
51	7	0	100	21	0	0.0475	0.1335	0.3225
52	7	0	100	22	1	0.0475	0.1335	0.3225
53	7	0	100	27	1	0.0475	0.1335	0.3225
54	8	0	150	20	0	0.1801	0.3445	0.5571

LOGISTIC REGRESSION ANALYSIS OF EXPERIMENT 148 = 5FU, CTX

'PROB' IS PREDICTED PROBABILITY OF SURVIVAL LONGER THAN 22.0 DAYS

ANIMAL	GROUP	X1	X2	SURVTIME	RESPONSE	_LOWER_	PROB	_UPPER_
55	8	0	150	20	0	0.1801	0.3445	0.5571
56	8	0	150	20	0	0.1801	0.3445	0.5571
57	8	0	150	21	0	0.1801	0.3445	0.5571
58	8	0	150	21	0	0.1801	0.3445	0.5571
59	8	0	150	23	1	0.1801	0.3445	0.5571
60	8	0	150	23	1	0.1801	0.3445	0.5571
61	8	0	150	23	1	0.1801	0.3445	0.5571
62	9	0	225	20	0	0.4606	0.6598	0.8150
63	9	0	225	21	0	0.4606	0.6598	0.8150
64	9	0	225	21	0	0.4606	0.6598	0.8150
65	9	0	225	22	1	0.4606	0.6598	0.8150
66	9	0	225	22	1	0.4606	0.6598	0.8150
67	9	0	225	29	1	0.4606	0.6598	0.8150
68	9	0	225	31	1	0.4606	0.6598	0.8150
69	9	0	225	34	1	0.4606	0.6598	0.8150
70	10	0	338	10	0	0.6260	0.8049	0.9105
71	10	0	338	20	0	0.6260	0.8049	0.9105
72	10	0	338	21	0	0.6260	0.8049	0.9105
73	10	0	338	21	0	0.6260	0.8049	0.9105
74	10	0	338	23	1	0.6260	0.8049	0.9105
75	10	0	338	32	1	0.6260	0.8049	0.9105
76	10	0	338	37	1	0.6260	0.8049	0.9105
77	10	0	338	41	1	0.6260	0.8049	0.9105
78	11	0	500	14	0	0.1979	0.4893	0.7881
79	11	0	500	18	0	0.1979	0.4893	0.7881
80	11	0	500	30	1	0.1979	0.4893	0.7881
81	11	0	500	34	1	0.1979	0.4893	0.7881
82	11	0	500	92	1	0.1979	0.4893	0.7881
83	11	0	500	103	1	0.1979	0.4893	0.7881
84	11	0	500	117	1	0.1979	0.4893	0.7881
85	12	100	100	117	1	0.3264	0.4568	0.5934
86	12	100	100	117	1	0.3264	0.4568	0.5934
87	12	100	100	17	0	0.3264	0.4568	0.5934
88	12	100	100	20	0	0.3264	0.4568	0.5934
89	12	100	100	20	0	0.3264	0.4568	0.5934
90	12	100	100	20	0	0.3264	0.4568	0.5934
91	12	100	100	22	1	0.3264	0.4568	0.5934
92	12	100	100	36	1	0.3264	0.4568	0.5934
93	13	100	150	9	0	0.5472	0.6647	0.7647
94	13	100	150	13	0	0.5472	0.6647	0.7647
95	13	100	150	23	1	0.5472	0.6647	0.7647
96	13	100	150	23	1	0.5472	0.6647	0.7647
97	13	100	150	23	1	0.5472	0.6647	0.7647
98	13	100	150	23	1	0.5472	0.6647	0.7647
99	13	100	150	26	1	0.5472	0.6647	0.7647
100	13	100	150	26	1	0.5472	0.6647	0.7647
101	14	100	225	20	0	0.7020	0.8077	0.8822
102	14	100	225	24	1	0.7020	0.8077	0.8822
103	14	100	225	26	1	0.7020	0.8077	0.8822
104	14	100	225	27	1	0.7020	0.8077	0.8822
105	14	100	225	27	1	0.7020	0.8077	0.8822
106	14	100	225	28	1	0.7020	0.8077	0.8822
107	14	100	225	30	1	0.7020	0.8077	0.8822
108	14	100	225	33	1	0.7020	0.8077	0.8822

LOGISTIC REGRESSION ANALYSIS OF EXPERIMENT 148 = 5FU, CTX

'PROB' IS PREDICTED PROBABILITY OF SURVIVAL LONGER THAN 22.0 DAYS

ANIMAL	GROUP	X1	X2	SURVTIME	RESPONSE	_LOWER_	PROB	_UPPER_
109	15	100	338	14	0	0.6759	0.7949	0.8781
110	15	100	338	14	0	0.6759	0.7949	0.8781
111	15	100	338	21	0	0.6759	0.7949	0.8781
112	15	100	338	23	1	0.6759	0.7949	0.8781
113	15	100	338	26	1	0.6759	0.7949	0.8781
114	15	100	338	35	1	0.6759	0.7949	0.8781
115	15	100	338	37	1	0.6759	0.7949	0.8781
116	15	100	338	46	1	0.6759	0.7949	0.8781
117	16	150	100	17	0	0.4011	0.5323	0.6591
118	16	150	100	20	0	0.4011	0.5323	0.6591
119	16	150	100	21	0	0.4011	0.5323	0.6591
120	16	150	100	21	0	0.4011	0.5323	0.6591
121	16	150	100	23	1	0.4011	0.5323	0.6591
122	16	150	100	23	1	0.4011	0.5323	0.6591
123	16	150	100	25	1	0.4011	0.5323	0.6591
124	16	150	100	27	1	0.4011	0.5323	0.6591
125	17	150	150	23	1	0.5702	0.6904	0.7894
126	17	150	150	23	1	0.5702	0.6904	0.7894
127	17	150	150	25	1	0.5702	0.6904	0.7894
128	17	150	150	25	1	0.5702	0.6904	0.7894
129	17	150	150	26	1	0.5702	0.6904	0.7894
130	17	150	150	26	1	0.5702	0.6904	0.7894
131	17	150	150	28	1	0.5702	0.6904	0.7894
132	17	150	150	30	1	0.5702	0.6904	0.7894
133	18	150	225	16	0	0.6685	0.7818	0.8642
134	18	150	225	20	0	0.6685	0.7818	0.8642
135	18	150	225	20	0	0.6685	0.7818	0.8642
136	18	150	225	23	1	0.6685	0.7818	0.8642
137	18	150	225	28	1	0.6685	0.7818	0.8642
138	18	150	225	30	1	0.6685	0.7818	0.8642
139	18	150	225	34	1	0.6685	0.7818	0.8642
140	18	150	225	37	1	0.6685	0.7818	0.8642
141	19	150	338	13	0	0.5190	0.6852	0.8146
142	19	150	338	15	0	0.5190	0.6852	0.8146
143	19	150	338	22	1	0.5190	0.6852	0.8146
144	19	150	338	28	1	0.5190	0.6852	0.8146
145	19	150	338	34	1	0.5190	0.6852	0.8146
146	19	150	338	41	1	0.5190	0.6852	0.8146
147	19	150	338	43	1	0.5190	0.6852	0.8146
148	20	225	100	18	0	0.3379	0.4753	0.6165
149	20	225	100	20	0	0.3379	0.4753	0.6165
150	20	225	100	20	0	0.3379	0.4753	0.6165
151	20	225	100	21	0	0.3379	0.4753	0.6165
152	20	225	100	21	0	0.3379	0.4753	0.6165
153	20	225	100	22	1	0.3379	0.4753	0.6165
154	20	225	100	23	1	0.3379	0.4753	0.6165
155	20	225	100	23	1	0.3379	0.4753	0.6165
156	21	225	150	117	1	0.4412	0.5736	0.6963
157	21	225	150	117	1	0.4412	0.5736	0.6963
158	21	225	150	117	1	0.4412	0.5736	0.6963
159	21	225	150	22	1	0.4412	0.5736	0.6963
160	21	225	150	23	1	0.4412	0.5736	0.6963
161	21	225	150	23	1	0.4412	0.5736	0.6963
162	21	225	150	26	1	0.4412	0.5736	0.6963

LOGISTIC REGRESSION ANALYSIS OF EXPERIMENT 148 - 5FU, CTX

'PROB' IS PREDICTED PROBABILITY OF SURVIVAL LONGER THAN 22.0 DAYS

ANIMAL	GROUP	X1	X2	SURVTIME	RESPONSE	_LOWER_	PROB	_UPPER_
163	21	225	150	41	1	0.4412	0.5736	0.6963
164	22	225	225	10	0	0.4457	0.5878	0.7166
165	22	225	225	14	0	0.4457	0.5878	0.7166
166	22	225	225	17	0	0.4457	0.5878	0.7166
167	22	225	225	17	0	0.4457	0.5878	0.7166
168	22	225	225	20	0	0.4457	0.5878	0.7166
169	22	225	225	27	1	0.4457	0.5878	0.7166
170	22	225	225	30	1	0.4457	0.5878	0.7166
171	23	225	338	13	0	0.1383	0.3166	0.5720
172	23	225	338	13	0	0.1383	0.3166	0.5720
173	23	225	338	14	0	0.1383	0.3166	0.5720
174	23	225	338	15	0	0.1383	0.3166	0.5720
175	23	225	338	18	0	0.1383	0.3166	0.5720
176	23	225	338	30	1	0.1383	0.3166	0.5720
177	23	225	338	37	1	0.1383	0.3166	0.5720
178	23	225	338	41	1	0.1383	0.3166	0.5720
179	24	338	100	14	0	0.0416	0.1204	0.3015
180	24	338	100	15	0	0.0416	0.1204	0.3015
181	24	338	100	16	0	0.0416	0.1204	0.3015
182	24	338	100	17	0	0.0416	0.1204	0.3015
183	24	338	100	20	0	0.0416	0.1204	0.3015
184	24	338	100	22	1	0.0416	0.1204	0.3015
185	24	338	100	23	1	0.0416	0.1204	0.3015
186	24	338	100	23	1	0.0416	0.1204	0.3015
187	25	338	150	14	0	0.0417	0.1181	0.2920
188	25	338	150	15	0	0.0417	0.1181	0.2920
189	25	338	150	16	0	0.0417	0.1181	0.2920
190	25	338	150	17	0	0.0417	0.1181	0.2920
191	25	338	150	18	0	0.0417	0.1181	0.2920
192	25	338	150	18	0	0.0417	0.1181	0.2920
193	25	338	150	18	0	0.0417	0.1181	0.2920
194	25	338	150	18	0	0.0417	0.1181	0.2920
195	26	338	225	14	0	0.0197	0.0705	0.2229
196	26	338	225	15	0	0.0197	0.0705	0.2229
197	26	338	225	15	0	0.0197	0.0705	0.2229
198	26	338	225	15	0	0.0197	0.0705	0.2229
199	26	338	225	17	0	0.0197	0.0705	0.2229
200	26	338	225	18	0	0.0197	0.0705	0.2229
201	26	338	225	20	0	0.0197	0.0705	0.2229
202	27	338	338	12	0	0.0010	0.0095	0.0857
203	27	338	338	12	0	0.0010	0.0095	0.0857
204	27	338	338	13	0	0.0010	0.0095	0.0857
205	27	338	338	14	0	0.0010	0.0095	0.0857
206	27	338	338	14	0	0.0010	0.0095	0.0857
207	27	338	338	14	0	0.0010	0.0095	0.0857
208	27	338	338	14	0	0.0010	0.0095	0.0857
209	27	338	338	17	0	0.0010	0.0095	0.0857

LOGISTIC REGRESSION ANALYSIS OF EXPERIMENT 148 = 5FU, CTX

GOODNESS-OF-FIT STATISTICS

GROUP	X1	X2	EXPECTED	OBSERVED	GRPCHI
1	0	0	0.04475	0	0.04500
2	100	0	0.30204	0	0.32146
3	150	0	0.89477	0	1.00744
4	225	0	1.18859	0	1.39599
5	338	0	0.45844	0	0.48631
6	500	0	0.00419	0	0.00419
7	0	100	1.06799	2	0.93864
8	0	150	2.75601	3	0.03295
9	0	225	5.27826	5	0.04312
10	0	338	6.43915	4	4.73561
11	0	500	3.42488	5	1.41836
12	100	100	3.65412	4	0.06027
13	100	150	5.31725	6	0.26143
14	100	225	6.46187	7	0.23309
15	100	338	6.35946	5	1.41716
16	150	100	4.25830	4	0.03350
17	150	150	5.52325	8	3.58738
18	150	225	6.25424	5	1.15263
19	150	338	4.79675	5	0.02736
20	225	100	3.80244	3	0.32274
21	225	150	4.58896	8	5.94651
22	225	225	4.11463	2	2.63655
23	225	338	2.53249	3	0.12628
24	338	100	0.96319	3	4.89667
25	338	150	0.94460	0	1.07106
26	338	225	0.49352	0	0.53096
27	338	338	0.07597	0	0.07670

LOGISTIC REGRESSION ANALYSIS OF EXPERIMENT 148 = 5FU, CTX

GOODNESS-OF-FIT STATISTICS

CHISQ=32.80934 P=0.04837441 DF=21 NUMGRPS=27

LOGISTIC REGRESSION ANALYSIS OF EXPERIMENT 148 = 5FU, CTX

CONTOUR PLOT OF CTX*_5FU

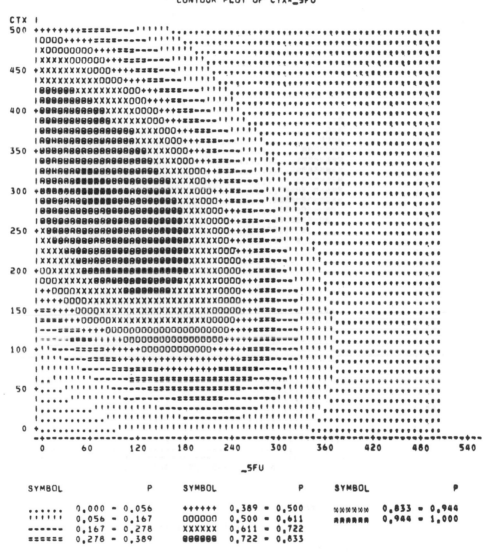

_5FU

SYMBOL	P	SYMBOL	P	SYMBOL	P
......	0.000 - 0.056	++++++	0.389 - 0.500	∞∞∞∞∞∞	0.833 - 0.944
!!!!!!	0.056 - 0.167	000000	0.500 - 0.611	⋒⋒⋒⋒⋒⋒	0.944 - 1.000
------	0.167 - 0.278	XXXXXX	0.611 - 0.722		
======	0.278 - 0.389	₿₿₿₿₿₿	0.722 - 0.833		

NOTE: 2365 OBS HIDDEN

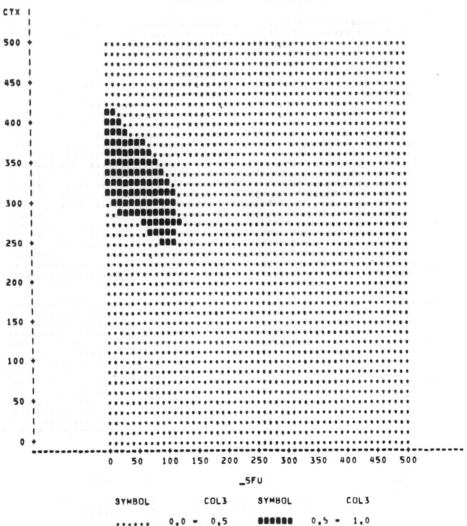

LOGISTIC REGRESSION ANALYSIS OF EXPERIMENT 148 = 5FU, CTX
ESTIMATED CONFIDENCE REGION
CONTOUR PLOT OF CTX*_5FU

_5FU

SYMBOL	COL3	SYMBOL	COL3
......	0.0 - 0.5	██████	0.5 - 1.0

NOTE: 511 OBS HIDDEN

MAIN PROGRAM FOR NELDER-MEAD SIMPLEX PROCEDURE

The following is a listing of the Fortran IV program used for
optimization of the function derived by using $\hat{\beta}$ from the logistic regression analysis or from the proportional hazards analysis (see below). It consists of a modified version of the main
program and subroutine given in [1]. These routines can be
used as they appear. However, the user must supply his own
double precision function subprogram to calculate the value of
the function to be optimized (see examples). Input required
is defined by comment cards found in the main program. An example of the input data cards appears after each of the function's subprograms. CNSTRN (1, K), K = 1, 2, has been added to
the program in order to constrain the search to the experimental region. Note that the parameters of the function, B(J),
J = 1, NP, are read in as data by the main program. The execution time for the program as applied to this example is approximately three seconds CPU time on an IBM-168, running MVS.

```
// EXEC FORTGCLG
//FORT.SYSIN DD *
C******************************************************************************C
C                                                                             C
C               MAIN PROGRAM FOR NELDER-MEAD SIMPLEX PROCEDURE                C
C                                                                             C
C******************************************************************************C
C                                                                             C
C                                                                             C
      DOUBLE PRECISION START(20),STEP(20),XMIN(20),
     1XSEC(20),YNEWLO,YSEC,REQMIN,DUMMY,FN,B(19),CNSTRN(4,2)
      COMMON B, CNSTRN, N
      DIMENSION TITLE(18), DRUG(4)
C                                                                             C
C         INPUT REQUIRED                                                      C
C                                                                             C
C         THE USER MUST SPECIFY THE FOLLOWING INPUT ON DATA CARDS:            C
C      TITLE          TITLE IDENTIFYING EXPERIMENT ANALYZED IN THIS RUN       C
C      ICOUNT         MAXIMUM NUMBER OF ITERATIONS ALLOWED                    C
C      N              NUMBER OF DRUGS IN THE COMBINATION                      C
C      NP             NUMBER OF PARAMETERS IN THE MODEL                       C
C      REQMIN         CONVERGENCE CRITERION                                   C
C      DRUG(I)        ITH DRUG IN THE COMBINATION                             C
C      CNSTRN(I,1)    MINIMUM VALUE OF ITH DRUG,  (DEFINES LOWER BOUND OF     C
C                     TREATMENT REGION TO BE EXPLORED)                        C
C      CNSTRN(I,2)    MAXIMUM VALUE OF ITH DRUG,  (DEFINES UPPER BOUND OF     C
C                     TREATMENT REGION TO BE EXPLORED)                        C
C      START(I)       STARTING VALUE OF ITH DRUG IN INITIAL SIMPLEX          C
C      STEP(I)        STEP SIZE FOR ITH DRUG FOR SIMPLEX SEARCH              C
C      B(J)           JTH PARAMETER IN FUNCTION TO BE OPTIMIZED              C
C                                                                             C
    1 READ(5,45,END=9999) TITLE
   45 FORMAT(18A4)
      READ(5,50) ICOUNT,N,NP,REQMIN
   50 FORMAT(3I5,D10.0)
      READ(5,53) (DRUG(I),CNSTRN(I,1),CNSTRN(I,2),I=1,N)
   53 FORMAT(A4,2D10.0)
      READ(5,55) (START(I),I=1,N)
   55 FORMAT(8D10.0)
      READ(5,55) (STEP(I),I=1,N)
      READ(5,55) (B(J),J=1,NP)
      WRITE(6,57) TITLE, ICOUNT,N,REQMIN,(DRUG(I),CNSTRN(I,1),CNSTRN(I,2
     1),START(I),STEP(I),I=1,N)
   57 FORMAT(1H1,18A4//1H0,33HMAXIMUM NO. ITERATIONS ALLOWED = ,I5/1H0,3
     11HNO. DRUGS IN THE COMBINATION = ,I5/1H0,24HCONVERGENCE CRITERION
     2= ,D10.3//1H0,4HDRUG,10X,18HREGION CONSTRAINTS,10X,14HSTARTING VAL
     3UE,10X,9HSTEP SIZE//(1H ,A4,8X,2F10.4,12X,F10.4,10X,F10.4)//)
C                                                                             C
      DO 60 I=1,N
      XMIN(I)=0.D0
      XSEC(I)=0.D0
   60 CONTINUE
      YNEWLO=0.D0
      YSEC=0.D0
C                                                                             C
C         CALL NELDER-MEAD SUBROUTINE                                         C
C                                                                             C
      CALL NELMIN(N,START,XMIN,XSEC,YNEWLO,YSEC,
     1REQMIN,STEP,ICOUNT)
C                                                                             C
```

```
C          OUTPUT FROM PROGRAM                                              C
C                                                                           C
      WRITE(6,65)ICOUNT
   65 FORMAT(1H0,//,I5,12H TRIALS USED/)
      WRITE(6,75)
   75 FORMAT(1H0,21X,9HESTIMATES/)
      WRITE(6,77)
   77 FORMAT(1H ,9HPARAMETER,3X,12HNEXT-TO-BEST,8X,
     14HBEST/)
      DO 79 I=1,N
   79 WRITE(6,80) I,XSEC(I),XMIN(I)
   80 FORMAT(1H0,I5,D20.7,D17.7)
      WRITE(6,82)
   82 FORMAT(1H0,6X,15HFUNCTION VALUES)
      WRITE(6,83)
   83 FORMAT(1H ,13H NEXT-TO-BEST,8X,4HBEST/)
      WRITE(6,84) YSEC,YNEWLO
   84 FORMAT(1H0,D14.7,D17.7)
 9999 CONTINUE
      STOP
      END
C---------------------------------------------------------------------------C
C                                                                           C
C     NELDER-MEAD SUBROUTINE                                                C
C                                                                           C
C---------------------------------------------------------------------------C
C                                                                           C
C                                                                           C
      SUBROUTINE NELMIN(N,START,XMIN,XSEC,YNEWLO,
     1YSEC,REQMIN,STEP,ICOUNT)
      DOUBLE PRECISION START(20),STEP(20),XMIN(20),
     1XSEC(20),YNEWLO,YSEC,REQMIN,P(20,21),PSTAR(20),
     2P2STAR(20),PBAR(20),Y(20),DN,Z,YLO,RCOEFF,
     3YSTAR,ECOEFF,Y2STAR,CCOEFF,FN,DABIT,DCHK,
     4COORD1,COORD2
      DATA RCOEFF/1.0D0/,ECOEFF/2.0D0/,CCOEFF/0.5D0/
      KCOUNT=ICOUNT
      ICOUNT=0
C                                                                           C
      IF( REQMIN .LE. 0.D0) ICOUNT=ICOUNT-1
      IF(N .LE. 0) ICOUNT=ICOUNT-10
      IF(N .GT. 20 ) ICOUNT=ICOUNT-10
      IF(ICOUNT .LT. 0) RETURN
C                                                                           C
      DABIT=2.04607D-35
      BIGNUM=1.0D38
      KONVGE=5
      XN=FLOAT(N)
      DN=DFLOAT(N)
      NN=N+1
C                                                                           C
C          CONSTRUCTION OF INITIAL SIMPLEX                                  C
C                                                                           C
 1001 DO 1 I=1,N
    1 P(I,NN)=START(I)
      Y(NN)=FN(START)
      ICOUNT=ICOUNT+1
      DO 2 J=1,N
      DCHK=START(J)
      START(J)=DCHK+STEP(J)
```

```
      DO 3 I=1,N
    3 P(I,J)=START(I)
      Y(J)=FN(START)
      ICOUNT=ICOUNT+1
    2 START(J) =DCHK
      WRITE (6,110) ((P(II,JJ),II=1,N),Y(JJ),JJ=1,NN)
  110 FORMAT(1H ,30HCOORDINATES OF INITIAL SIMPLEX,10X,15HFUNCTION VALUE
     1S//(2X,2(3X,F10.4),14X,D12.5)/)
C
C         SIMPLEX CONSTRUCTION COMPLETE
C
C         FIND HIGHEST AND LOWEST Y VALUES
C         YNEWLO (Y(IHI)) INDICATES THE VERTEX OF
C         THE SIMPLEX TO BE REPLACED
C
 1000 YLO=Y(1)
      YNEWLO=YLO
      ILO=1
      IHI=1
      DO 5 I=2,NN
      IF(Y(I) .GE. YLO) GO TO 4
      YLO=Y(I)
      ILO=I
    4 IF(Y(I) .LE. YNEWLO) GO TO 5
      YNEWLO=Y(I)
      IHI=I
    5 CONTINUE
C
C         PERFORM CONVERGENCE CHECKS ON FUNCTION
C
      DCHK=(YNEWLO+DABIT)/(YLO+DABIT)-1.D0
      IF(DABS(DCHK) .LT. REQMIN) GO TO 900
      KONVGF=KONVGF-1
      IF(KONVGE .NE. 0) GO TO 2020
      KONVGE=5
C
C         CHECK CONVERGENCE OF COORDINATES ONLY
C         EVERY 5 SIMPLEXES
C
      DO 2015 I=1,N
      COORD1=P(I,1)
      COORD2=COORD1
      DO 2010 J=2,NN
      IF(P(I,J) .GE. COORD1) GO TO 2005
      COORD1=P(I,J)
 2005 IF(P(I,J) .LE. COORD2) GO TO 2010
      COORD2=P(I,J)
 2010 CONTINUE
      DCHK=(COORD2+DABIT)/(COORD1+DABIT)-1.D0
      IF(DABS(DCHK) .GT. REQMIN) GO TO 2020
 2015 CONTINUE
      GO TO 900
 2020 IF(ICOUNT .GE. KCOUNT) GO TO 900
C
C         CALCULATE PBAR, THE CENTROID OF THE
C         SIMPLEX VERTICES EXCEPTING THAT WITH
C         Y VALUE YNEWLO
C
      DO 7 I=1,N
      Z=0.0D0
```

```
          DO 6 J=1,NN
        6 Z=Z+P(I,J)
          Z=Z-P(I,IHI)
        7 PBAR(I)=Z/DN
C                                                                    C
C             REFLECTION THROUGH THE CENTROID                        C
C                                                                    C
          DO 8 I=1,N
        8 PSTAR(I)=(1.0D0+RCOEFF)*PBAR(I)-RCOEFF*P(I,IHI)
          YSTAR=FN(PSTAR)
          ICOUNT=ICOUNT+1
          IF(YSTAR .GE. YLO) GO TO 12
          IF(ICOUNT .GE. KCOUNT) GO TO 19
C                                                                    C
C             SUCCESSFUL REFLECTION, SO EXTENSION                    C
C                                                                    C
          DO 9 I=1,N
        9 P2STAR(I)=ECOEFF*PSTAR(I)+(1.0D0-ECOEFF)*PBAR(I)
          Y2STAR=FN(P2STAR)
          ICOUNT=ICOUNT+1
C                                                                    C
C             RETAIN EXTENSION OR CONTRACTION                        C
C                                                                    C
          IF(Y2STAR .GE. YSTAR) GO TO 19
       10 DO 11 I=1,N
       11 P(I,IHI)=P2STAR(I)
          Y(IHI)=Y2STAR
          GO TO 1000
C                                                                    C
C             NO EXTENSION                                           C
C                                                                    C
       12 L=0
          DO 13 I=1,NN
          IF(Y(I) .GT. YSTAR) L=L+1
       13 CONTINUE
          IF(L .GT. 1) GO TO 19
          IF(L .EQ. 0) GO TO 15
C                                                                    C
C             CONTRACTION ON THE REFLECTION SIDE OF THE              C
C             CENTROID                                               C
C                                                                    C
          DO 14 I=1,N
       14 P(I,IHI)=PSTAR(I)
          Y(IHI)=YSTAR
C                                                                    C
C             CONTRACTION ON THE Y(IHI) SIDE OF THE CENTROID         C
C                                                                    C
       15 IF(ICOUNT .GE. KCOUNT) GO TO 900
          DO 16 I=1,N
       16 P2STAR(I)=CCOEFF*P(I,IHI)+(1.0D0-CCOEFF)*PBAR(I)
          Y2STAR=FN(P2STAR)
          ICOUNT=ICOUNT+1
          IF(Y2STAR .LT. Y(IHI)) GO TO 10
C                                                                    C
C             CONTRACT THE WHOLE SIMPLEX                             C
C                                                                    C
          DO 18 J=1,NN
          DO 17 I=1,N
          P(I,J)=(P(I,J)+P(I,ILO))*0.5D0
       17 XMIN(I)=P(I,J)
```

```
          Y(J)=FN(XMIN)
       18 CONTINUE
          ICOUNT=ICOUNT+NN
          IF(ICOUNT .LT. KCOUNT) GO TO 1000
          GO TO 900
C                                                                    C
C             RETAIN REFLECTION                                      C
C                                                                    C
       19 CONTINUE
          DO 20 I=1,N
       20 P(I,IHI)=PSTAR(I)
          Y(IHI)=YSTAR
          GO TO 1000
C                                                                    C
C             SELECT THE TWO BEST FUNCTION VALUES (YNEWLO            C
C             AND YSEC) AND THEIR COORDS, (XMIN AND SXEC)            C
C                                                                    C
      900 DO 23 J=1,NN
          DO 22 I=1,N
       22 XMIN(I)=P(I,J)
          Y(J)=FN(XMIN)
       23 CONTINUE
          YNEWLO=BIGNUM
          DO 24 J=1,NN
          IF(Y(J) .GE. YNEWLO) GO TO 24
          YNEWLO=Y(J)
          IBEST=J
       24 CONTINUE
          Y(IBEST)=BIGNUM
          YSEC=BIGNUM
          DO 25 J=1,NN
          IF(Y(J) .GE. YSEC) GO TO 25
          YSEC=Y(J)
          ISEC=J
       25 CONTINUE
          DO 26 I=1,N
          XMIN(I)=P(I,IBEST)
          XSEC(I)=P(I,ISEC)
       26 CONTINUE
          RETURN
          END
```

The subsequent listing is an example of the Fortran IV double precision function subprogram supplied by the user. In the card deck, it and the data cards follow the Nelder-Mead subroutine immediately. The name of the function is FN. It is called by the Nelder-Mead subroutine and returns the value calculated (for the logistic function, in this example) to that subroutine. The user should note that the Nelder-Mead routine is for function minimization. If it is desired to maximize a function, f($\underline{x}$), the user should work with -f($\underline{x}$). Following the function subprogram, the data cards required and appropriate JCL are listed in their proper locations.

```
C------------------------------------------------------------------------C
C                                                                        C
C     PROGRAM 'FUNCTION' - CALCULATES VALUE OF FUNCTION TO BE OPTIMIZED   C
C                         (LOGISTIC EXAMPLE)                              C
C                                                                        C
C------------------------------------------------------------------------C
C                                                                        C
C                                                                        C
      DOUBLE PRECISION FUNCTION FN(X)
      DOUBLE PRECISION X(4),B(19),CNSTRN(4,2),XPB
      COMMON B,CNSTRN,N
      DO 5 I=1,N
      IF (X(I).LT.CNSTRN(I,1)) GO TO 10
      IF (X(I).GT.CNSTRN(I,2)) GO TO 10
    5 CONTINUE
C                                                                        C
C        CALCULATION OF VALUE OF FUNCTION TO BE OPTIMIZED FOLLOWS         C
C                                                                        C
      XPB = B(1) + B(2)*X(1) + B(3)*X(2) + B(4)*X(1)*X(1) + B(5)*X(2)*X(
     12) + B(6)*X(1)*X(2)
      FN = 1 / (1 + DEXP(-XPB))
      FN=-FN
      RETURN
   10 FN=1.0D38
      RETURN
      END
//GO.SYSIN DD *
```

DATA CARDS ARE PLACED HERE, PUNCHED AS FOLLOWS:

```
EXP 148 - 5FU, CTX                    LOGISTIC PARAMETERS
   800    2    6 .00000001
5FU         0.0         500.
CTX         0.0         500.
         60.         300.
         .01          .01
-5.18048780.031639010.03880772-.00007277-.00005707-.00007392
```

The following is the computer output obtained from execution of the preceding program and subprograms. In order of their appearance are the coordinates of the initial simplex and the function value at each of those points, the number of trials used, the best and next-to-best estimates of the coordinates of the optimum point (drug combination) and the values of the function at those points. The optimal combination estimated for this experiment is a dose of 66.6 mg/kg of 5-FU and 296.8 mg/kg of CTX with an associated estimated maximum probability of 0.8366551.

```
EXP 148 - 5FU, CTX                      LOGISTIC PARAMETERS

MAXIMUM NO. ITERATIONS ALLOWED =    800
NO. DRUGS IN THE COMBINATION =      2
CONVERGENCE CRITERION =  0.100D-07
```

DRUG	REGION CONSTRAINTS		STARTING VALUE	STEP SIZE
5FU	0.0	500.0000	60.0000	0.0100
CTX	0.0	500.0000	300.0000	0.0100

COORDINATES OF INITIAL SIMPLEX		FUNCTION VALUES
60.0100	300.0000	-0.83635D 00
60.0000	300.0100	-0.83635D 00
60.0000	300.0000	-0.83635D 00

```
   85 TRIALS USED

                      ESTIMATES
PARAMETER    NEXT-TO-BEST        BEST

    1        0.6663898D 02    0.6662761D 02
    2        0.2968493D 03    0.2968388D 03
        FUNCTION VALUES
  NEXT-TO-BEST        BEST

-0.8366551D 00    -0.8366551D 00
```

PROPORTIONAL HAZARDS ANALYSIS

The SAS program which follows performs the proportional hazards
analysis on a two-drug combination experiment. Also, it plots
contours of constant response for the two drugs, plots the estimated confidence region for the optimal combination of the two,
and calculates the Spearman rank-order correlation coefficient
of the estimated relative hazard and the median survival time
for the treatment groups. The proportional hazards analysis
utilizes the PHGLM procedure. Definitions for the six "MACRO"s,
explained on comment cards given initially in the listing, must
be furnished by the user. Data is read from cards which should
follow the "CARDS" statement. Cards should be punched as shown
below, each value being separated from the next by at least one
blank. The example cards are taken from the data in Table A.1.
Each line represents one card, which contains all the input information for one subject: group number, event indicator (1 for
dead, 0 for censored), survival time, dose of first drug, dose
of second drug.

1	1	10	0	0
1	1	10	0	0
1	1	11	0	0
1	1	11	0	0
:	:	:	:	:
27	1	14	338	338
27	1	14	338	338
27	1	14	338	338
27	1	17	338	338

On an IBM-168, running MVS, SPU time used for this experiment
was approximately one minute.

```
// EXEC SAS,REGION=512K
*********************************************************************************
*
*     PROPORTIONAL HAZARDS ANALYSIS AND DENSITY PLOT
*
*********************************************************************************
*
*THE FOLLOWING MACRO DEFINITIONS ARE SET BY THE USER FOR EACH RUN:
*   NAMETITL    TITLE IDENTIFYING EXPERIMENT ANALYZED IN THIS RUN
*   TERMS       LIST OF INDEPENDENT VARIABLES IN THE MODEL
*   DRUG1       NAME OF VARIABLE 'X1' WHICH IS THE FIRST DRUG IN THE COMBINATION
*   DRUG2       NAME OF VARIABLE 'X2' WHICH IS THE SECOND DRUG IN THE COMBINATION
*   HORIZMAX    A NUMBER <= HIGHEST DOSAGE LEVEL OF DRUG1,  USED TO DEFINE RANGE
*               OF HORIZONTAL AXIS FOR PLOT
*   VERTMAX     A NUMBER <= HIGHEST DOSAGE LEVEL OF DRUG2,  USED TO DEFINE RANGE
*               OF VERTICAL AXIS FOR PLOT
*
MACRO NAMETITL EXPERIMENT 148 - 5FU, CTX%
MACRO DRUG1 _5FU%
MACRO DRUG2 CTX%
MACRO TERMS X1 X2 X1SQ X2SQ X1X2%
MACRO HORIZMAX 500%
MACRO VERTMAX 500%
*
*----------------------------------------------------------------------------
*
*     PROPORTIONAL HAZARDS ANALYSIS
*
*----------------------------------------------------------------------------
*
TITLE PROPORTIONAL HAZARDS ANALYSIS OF NAMETITL;
*
*READ DATA IN FOLLOWING STEP:
*   GROUP       TREATMENT GROUP TO WHICH SUBJECT BELONGS
*   CENSOR      EVENT INDICATOR,  '0' INDICATES SUBJECT STILL ALIVE AT END OF
*               STUDY,  '1' INDICATES THAT SUBJECT DIED.
*   SURVTIME    TIME TO FAILURE
*   X1          DOSE OF FIRST DRUG IN THE COMBINATION
*   X2          DOSE OF SECOND DRUG IN THE COMBINATION
*
DATA EXP;
  INPUT GROUP CENSOR SURVTIME X1 X2;
DUM=1;
*
*   CALCULATE VALUES OF REMAINING INDEPENDENT VARIABLES IN MODEL
*
  X1SQ = X1*X1;
  X2SQ = X2*X2;
  X1X2 = X1*X2;
  CARDS;
*
*DATA CARDS GO HERE
*
DATA MODIFIED;
  SET EXP;
  ANIMAL = _N_;
PROC PRINT; VAR GROUP X1 X2 SURVTIME CENSOR; ID ANIMAL;
*
*'PROC SORT' USED TO SORT OBSERVATIONS BY SURVIVAL TIME IN DESCENDING ORDER
*               AS REQUIRED BY 'PROC PHGLM'
```

```
*                                                                          |
PROC SORT; BY DESCENDING SURVTIME;
*                                                                          |
*'PROC PHGLM' USED TO PERFORM ANALYSIS AND TO OUTPUT ESTIMATES AND COVARIANCE |
*              MATRIX TO DATASET 'BETAS'                                    |
*MODEL DEFINED IN MACRO 'TERMS' AT BEGINNING OF PROGRAM                     |
*                                                                          |
PROC PHGLM OUTPUT OUT=BETAS PRINTC;
  EVENT CENSOR;
  MODEL SURVTIME = TERMS;
  TITLE4 X1=DRUG1 X2=DRUG2;
*                                                                          |
*'PROC MEANS' USED TO CALCULATE AND OUTPUT TO DATASET MINIMUM VALUES AND    |
*              RANGES OF DOSAGE LEVELS OF DRUGS                             |
*                                                                          |
PROC MEANS DATA=MODIFIED NOPRINT; VAR X1 X2;
  OUTPUT OUT=DIMENS MIN=MIN_X1 MIN_X2 RANGE=RANGE_X1 RANGE_X2;
*                                                                          |
*--------------------------------------------------------------------------|
*                                                                          |
*     PLOT OF CONTOURS OF CONSTANT RESPONSE FOR COMBINATION OF TWO DRUGS    |
*                                                                          |
*--------------------------------------------------------------------------|
*                                                                          |
DATA BETANEW;
  MERGE BETAS DIMENS;
*                                                                          |
*DATA STEP 'PLOTIT' AND MACRO 'PROCESS' GENERATE THE GRID OF OBSERVATIONS FOR |
*              THE PLOT AND CALCULATE THE ESTIMATED PROBABILITY OF SURVIVAL AT |
*              EACH POINT                                                   |
*                                                                          |
MACRO PROCESS
  X = MIN_X1 + IO * RANGE_X1;
  Y = MIN_X2 + JO * RANGE_X2;
  XPB= X1*X + X2*Y + X1SQ*(X**2) + X2SQ*(Y**2) + X1X2*X*Y;
  IF XPB>1.0 THEN XPB=1.0;
  P = -XPB;
  FORMAT P 5.3;
  OUTPUT;
%
DATA PLOTIT;
  SET BETANEW;
  IF _N_=1;
  DO I = 0 TO 100;
    IO = I/100;
    DO J = 0 TO 50;
      JO = J/50;
    PROCESS;
    END;
  END;
DATA REDUCED;
  SET PLOTIT;
  IF X<=HORIZMAX AND Y<=VERTMAX;
  RENAME X=DRUG1 Y=DRUG2;
PROC PLOT;
  PLOT DRUG2*DRUG1=P / CONTOUR=10;
  TITLE2  ;
```

```
*                                                                          :
*-------------------------------------------------------------------------:
*                                                                          :
*      PLOT OF ESTIMATED CONFIDENCE REGION FOR THE OPTIMUM COMBINATION OF  :
*              TWO DRUGS                                                    :
*                                                                          :
*-------------------------------------------------------------------------:
*                                                                          :
PROC MATRIX;
FETCH BIGMAT DATA=BETANEW;
NC = NCOL(BIGMAT);
NR=NROW(BIGMAT);
XC = NC - 4;
B = BIGMAT(1,1:XC);
V = BIGMAT(2:NR,1:XC);
MIN_X1 = BIGMAT(1,6);
MIN_X2 = BIGMAT(1,7);
RANGE_X1 = BIGMAT(1,8);
RANGE_X2 = BIGMAT(1,9);
MAX_X1 = MIN_X1 + RANGE_X1;
MAX_X2 = MIN_X2 + RANGE_X2;
ZZ = MIN_X1//MIN_X2//0;
ZZ = ZZ';
DO X1 = MIN_X1 TO MAX_X1 BY RANGE_X1 #/50;
  DO X2 = MIN_X2 TO MAX_X2 BY RANGE_X2 #/50;
    L1   = B(1,1) + 2*B(1,3)*X1 + B(1,5)*X2;
    L2   = B(1,2) + 2*B(1,4)*X2 + B(1,5)*X1;
    VAR1 = V(1,1) + 4*(X1**2)*V(3,3) + (X2**2)*V(5,5) + 4*X1*V(1,3)
           + 2*X2*V(1,5) + 4*X1*X2*V(3,5);
    VAR2 = V(2,2) + 4*(X2**2)*V(4,4) + (X1**2)*V(5,5) + 4*X2*V(2,4)
           + 2*X1*V(2,5) + 4*X1*X2*V(4,5);
    VAR12 = V(1,2) + 2*X2*V(1,4) + X1*V(1,5) + 2*X1*V(2,3) + 4*X1*X2*V(3,4)
           + 2*(X1**2)*V(3,5) + X2*V(2,5) + 2*(X2**2)*V(4,5) + X1*X2*V(5,5);
    L = L1//L2;
    VA = VAR1//VAR12;
    VB = VAR12//VAR2;
    VCVL = VA'//VB';
    Y = L'*INV(VCVL)*L;
    W = 0;  IF Y<5.99 THEN W=1;
    Z = X1//X2//W;
    ZZ = ZZ//Z';
  END;
END;
OUTPUT B OUT=ESTS (RENAME=(COL1=B1 COL2=B2 COL3=B11 COL4=B22 COL5=B12));
OUTPUT ZZ OUT=NEW (RENAME=(COL1=DRUG1 COL2=DRUG2));
PROC PLOT;
PLOT DRUG2*DRUG1=COL3 / CONTOUR=2;
TITLE3 ESTIMATED CONFIDENCE REGION;
*                                                                          :
*-------------------------------------------------------------------------:
*                                                                          :
*      CORRELATION COEFFICIENT                                             :
*                                                                          :
*-------------------------------------------------------------------------:
*                                                                          :
*THIS STEP CALCULATES THE CORRELATION BETWEEN THE RANKS OF THE RELATIVE HAZARD :
*              FOR THE TREATMENT GROUPS AND THE RANKS OF THE MEDIAN SURVIVAL :
*              TIME FOR THE TREATMENT GROUPS                               :
*                                                                          :
DATA BHAT; SET ESTS;
```

```
DUM=1;
DATA EXPSRT;
  SET EXP;
PROC SORT; BY GROUP SURVTIME;
  PROC UNIVARIATE NOPRINT; VAR SURVTIME; BY GROUP;
    OUTPUT OUT=MEDN MEDIAN=MED;
DATA ONE;
  SET EXPSRT; BY GROUP;
  IF FIRST.GROUP;
DATA TWO;
  MERGE ONE MEDN; BY GROUP;
DATA CORRTEST;
  MERGE TWO BHAT; BY DUM;
Y = EXP(B1*X1 + B2*X2 + B11*X1*X1 + B22*X2*X2 + B12*X1*X2);
PROC PRINT; VAR X1 X2 Y MED;
  ID GROUP;
  TITLE3 Y = RELATIVE HAZARD   MED = MEDIAN;
PROC CORR SPEARMAN;
  VAR MED Y;
//
```

The computer output from the preceding program, run on the data in Table A.1, is as follows.

PROPORTIONAL HAZARDS ANALYSIS OF EXPERIMENT 148 - 5FU, CTX

ANIMAL	GROUP	X1	X2	SURVTIME	CENSOR
1	1	0	0	10	1
2	1	0	0	10	1
3	1	0	0	11	1
4	1	0	0	11	1
5	1	0	0	11	1
6	1	0	0	11	1
7	1	0	0	11	1
8	1	0	0	12	1
9	2	100	0	13	1
10	2	100	0	14	1
11	2	100	0	14	1
12	2	100	0	15	1
13	2	100	0	15	1
14	3	150	0	14	1
15	3	150	0	14	1
16	3	150	0	14	1
17	3	150	0	15	1
18	3	150	0	15	1
19	3	150	0	15	1
20	3	150	0	15	1
21	3	150	0	17	1
22	4	225	0	13	1
23	4	225	0	14	1
24	4	225	0	15	1
25	4	225	0	15	1
26	4	225	0	15	1
27	4	225	0	15	1
28	4	225	0	15	1
29	4	225	0	16	1
30	5	338	0	16	1
31	5	338	0	16	1
32	5	338	0	16	1
33	5	338	0	17	1
34	5	338	0	17	1
35	5	338	0	17	1
36	5	338	0	18	1
37	5	338	0	18	1
38	6	500	0	13	1
39	6	500	0	13	1
40	6	500	0	16	1
41	6	500	0	17	1
42	6	500	0	17	1
43	6	500	0	17	1
44	6	500	0	17	1
45	6	500	0	18	1
46	7	0	100	10	1
47	7	0	100	20	1
48	7	0	100	20	1
49	7	0	100	20	1
50	7	0	100	20	1
51	7	0	100	21	1
52	7	0	100	22	1
53	7	0	100	27	1
54	8	0	150	20	1
55	8	0	150	20	1
56	8	0	150	20	1

PROPORTIONAL HAZARDS ANALYSIS OF EXPERIMENT 148 - 5FU, CTX

ANIMAL	GROUP	X1	X2	SURVTIME	CENSOR
57	8	0	150	21	1
58	8	0	150	21	1
59	8	0	150	23	1
60	8	0	150	23	1
61	8	0	150	23	1
62	9	0	225	20	1
63	9	0	225	21	1
64	9	0	225	21	1
65	9	0	225	22	1
66	9	0	225	22	1
67	9	0	225	29	1
68	9	0	225	31	1
69	9	0	225	34	1
70	10	0	338	10	1
71	10	0	338	20	1
72	10	0	338	21	1
73	10	0	338	21	1
74	10	0	338	23	1
75	10	0	338	32	1
76	10	0	338	37	1
77	10	0	338	41	1
78	11	0	500	14	1
79	11	0	500	18	1
80	11	0	500	30	1
81	11	0	500	34	1
82	11	0	500	92	1
83	11	0	500	103	1
84	11	0	500	117	1
85	12	100	100	117	0
86	12	100	100	117	0
87	12	100	100	17	1
88	12	100	100	20	1
89	12	100	100	20	1
90	12	100	100	20	1
91	12	100	100	22	1
92	12	100	100	36	1
93	13	100	150	9	1
94	13	100	150	13	1
95	13	100	150	23	1
96	13	100	150	23	1
97	13	100	150	23	1
98	13	100	150	23	1
99	13	100	150	26	1
100	13	100	150	26	1
101	14	100	225	20	1
102	14	100	225	24	1
103	14	100	225	26	1
104	14	100	225	27	1
105	14	100	225	27	1
106	14	100	225	28	1
107	14	100	225	30	1
108	14	100	225	33	1
109	15	100	338	14	1
110	15	100	338	14	1
111	15	100	338	21	1
112	15	100	338	23	1

PROPORTIONAL HAZARDS ANALYSIS OF EXPERIMENT 148 = 5FU, CTX

ANIMAL	GROUP	X1	X2	SURVTIME	CENSOR
113	15	100	338	26	1
114	15	100	338	35	1
115	15	100	338	37	1
116	15	100	338	46	1
117	16	150	100	17	1
118	16	150	100	20	1
119	16	150	100	21	1
120	16	150	100	21	1
121	16	150	100	23	1
122	16	150	100	23	1
123	16	150	100	25	1
124	16	150	100	27	1
125	17	150	150	23	1
126	17	150	150	23	1
127	17	150	150	25	1
128	17	150	150	25	1
129	17	150	150	26	1
130	17	150	150	26	1
131	17	150	150	28	1
132	17	150	150	30	1
133	18	150	225	16	1
134	18	150	225	20	1
135	18	150	225	20	1
136	18	150	225	23	1
137	18	150	225	28	1
138	18	150	225	30	1
139	18	150	225	34	1
140	18	150	225	37	1
141	19	150	338	13	1
142	19	150	338	15	1
143	19	150	338	22	1
144	19	150	338	28	1
145	19	150	338	34	1
146	19	150	338	41	1
147	19	150	338	43	1
148	20	225	100	18	1
149	20	225	100	20	1
150	20	225	100	20	1
151	20	225	100	21	1
152	20	225	100	21	1
153	20	225	100	22	1
154	20	225	100	23	1
155	20	225	100	23	1
156	21	225	150	117	0
157	21	225	150	117	0
158	21	225	150	117	0
159	21	225	150	22	1
160	21	225	150	23	1
161	21	225	150	23	1
162	21	225	150	26	1
163	21	225	150	41	1
164	22	225	225	10	1
165	22	225	225	14	1
166	22	225	225	17	1
167	22	225	225	17	1
168	22	225	225	20	1

PROPORTIONAL HAZARDS ANALYSIS OF EXPERIMENT 148 - 5FU, CTX

ANIMAL	GROUP	X1	X2	SURVTIME	CENSOR
169	22	225	225	27	1
170	22	225	225	30	1
171	23	225	338	13	1
172	23	225	338	13	1
173	23	225	338	14	1
174	23	225	338	15	1
175	23	225	338	18	1
176	23	225	338	30	1
177	23	225	338	37	1
178	23	225	338	41	1
179	24	338	100	14	1
180	24	338	100	15	1
181	24	338	100	16	1
182	24	338	100	17	1
183	24	338	100	20	1
184	24	338	100	22	1
185	24	338	100	23	1
186	24	338	100	23	1
187	25	338	150	14	1
188	25	338	150	15	1
189	25	338	150	16	1
190	25	338	150	17	1
191	25	338	150	18	1
192	25	338	150	18	1
193	25	338	150	18	1
194	25	338	150	18	1
195	26	338	225	14	1
196	26	338	225	15	1
197	26	338	225	15	1
198	26	338	225	15	1
199	26	338	225	17	1
200	26	338	225	18	1
201	26	338	225	20	1
202	27	338	338	12	1
203	27	338	338	12	1
204	27	338	338	13	1
205	27	338	338	14	1
206	27	338	338	14	1
207	27	338	338	14	1
208	27	338	338	14	1
209	27	338	338	17	1

PROPORTIONAL HAZARDS ANALYSIS OF EXPERIMENT 148 - 5FU, CTX

X1= _5FU X2= CTX

PROPORTIONAL HAZARDS GENERAL LINEAR MODEL PROCEDURE

DEPENDENT VARIABLE: SURVTIME

EVENT INDICATOR: CENSOR

209 OBSERVATIONS
204 UNCENSORED OBSERVATIONS
211 EQUIVALENT SAMPLE SIZE WITH NO CENSORING
  0 OBSERVATIONS DELETED DUE TO MISSING VALUES

-2 LOG LIKELIHOOD FOR MODEL CONTAINING NO VARIABLES= 1836.59

CONVERGENCE OBTAINED IN 5 ITERATIONS.   D=0.346.
MAX ABSOLUTE DERIVATIVE=0.1612D-02.   -2 LOG L= 1727.80.
MODEL CHI-SQUARE= 108.79 WITH   5 D.F.   P=0.0   .

VARIABLE	BETA	STD. ERROR	CHI-SQUARE	P	D
X1	-0.01447346	0.00226688	40.77	0.0000	0.165
X2	-0.02640617	0.00301408	76.75	0.0	0.271
X1SQ	0.00002306	0.00000418	30.48	0.0000	0.129
X2SQ	0.00003754	0.00000519	52.33	0.0000	0.203
X1X2	0.00005099	0.00000601	71.97	0.0000	0.259

PROPORTIONAL HAZARDS ANALYSIS OF EXPERIMENT 148 - 5FU, CTX

X1= _5FU X2= CTX

PROPORTIONAL HAZARDS GENERAL LINEAR MODEL PROCEDURE

DEPENDENT VARIABLE: SURVTIME

EVENT INDICATOR: CENSOR

COVARIANCE MATRIX OF ESTIMATES

	X1	X2	X1SQ	X2SQ	X1X2
X1	.00000513874	.00000256827	-8.78427E-09	-2.63206E-09	-9.68448E-09
X2	.00000256827	.00000908467	-2.05232E-09	-1.49422E-08	-1.38798E-08
X1SQ	-8.78427E-09	-2.05232E-09	1.74448E-11	7.78749E-13	1.28183F-11
X2SQ	-2.63206E-09	-1.49422E-08	7.78749E-13	2.69316E-11	1.94057E-11
X1X2	-9.68448E-09	-1.38798E-08	1.28183E-11	1.94057E-11	3.61239E-11

PROPORTIONAL HAZARDS ANALYSIS OF EXPERIMENT 148 = 5FU, CTX

CONTOUR PLOT OF CTX*_5FU

```
CTX |
    |
500 +■■888888XXXXXX000000+++++====----!!!!
    |■■888888888XXXXXX00000++++++=====----!!!  ............................
    |■■88888888888888XXXXX0000000++++====----  ...........................
    |■■8888888888888888XXXXXX00000++++++====----   .........................
450 +■■88888888888888888XXXXX00000+++++++=====----!!!  ........................
    |■■888888888888888888XXXXXX0000000+++++====-----!!!  .....................
    |■■88888888888888888888XXXXXX00000++++++====-----!!!  ....................
    |■■888888888888888888888XXXXXX00000++++++=====-----!!!  ..................
400 +■■888888888888888888888888XXXXXX000000++++++=====------!!!!  .............
    |■■8888888888888888888888888XXXXXX000000++++++=====-----!!!!  ............
    |■■■888888888888888888888888888XXXXXX00000+++++====----!!!!  .............
    |■■■8888888888888888888888888888XXXXXX000000+++++====----!!!!  ...........
350 +■■■8888888888888888888888888888XXXXXX00000++++++=====----!!!!  ..........
    |■■■■88888888888888888888888888888XXXXXX000000+++++=====----!!!  .........
    |■■■■88888888888888888888888888888888XXXXXX000000++++++=====----!!!!  .....
    |■■■■■8888888888888888888888888888888XXXXXX00000++++++=====-----!!!!  .....
300 +■■■■■888888888888888888888888888888888XXXXXX000000++++++=====----!!!!  ...
    |■■■■■888888888888888888888888888888888888XXXXXXX00000++++++=====-----!!!!  .
    |■■■■■■88888888888888888888888888888888888XXXXX0000000+++++=====----!!!!  .
250 +■■■■■■888888888888888888888888888888888888XXXXXX000000+++++=====----!!!!
    |■■■■■■■888888888888888888888888888888888888XXXXXX000000+++++++=====----!!!!
    |■■■■■■■■88888888888888888888888888888888888888XXXXXXX000000++++++=====----
    |■■■■■■■■■8888888888888888888888888888888888888XXXXXX0000000+++++=====-----
200 +■■■■■■88888888888888888888888888888888888888888XXXXXXX000000+++++++=====---
    |■8888888888888888888888888888888888888888888XXXXXXX0000000++++++=====---
    |■888888888888888888888888888888888888888888888XXXXXXXXX000000++++++=====
    |■8888888888888888888888888888888888888888888888XXXXXXXXX0000000++++++=====
150 +■8888888888888888888888888888888888888888888888888XXXXXXXXX00000000+++++++====
    |XXX88888888888888888888888888888888888888888888888888XXXXXXXXX00000000++++++==
    |XXXXXXXXX8888888888888888888888888888888888888888888XXXXXXXXX000000000+++++==
    |XXXXXXXXXXXX8888888888888888888888888888888888888888XXXXXXXXX00000000+++++==
100 +0000XXXXXXXX8888888888888888888888888888888XXXXXXXXXXXXXX00000000UUU+++++++++
    |0000000XXXXXXXXXXXXXXXXX8888888888888888XXXXXXXXXXXXXXX000000000++++++++
    |++0000000000000XXXXXXXXXXXXXXXXXXXXXXXXXXXXXXXXXX0000000000+++++++
    |++++++0000000000000XXXXXXXXXXXXXXXXXXXXXXXXXXXXXXX0000000000+++++++
 50 +++++++++00000000000000XXXXXXXXXXXXXXXXXXXXXXXXXX00000000000++++++
    |====++++++++0000000000000XXXXXXXXXXXXXXXXXXXXXX00000000000+++++++
    |========+++++++0000000000000000XXXXXXXX0000000000000000++++++
    |-----=======+++++++0000000000000000000XXXXXXX00000000000000000++++++
  0 +------=======+++++++++000000000000000000000000000000000000++++++
    -+---------+---------+---------+---------+---------+---------+---------+---------+---------+--
     0        60       120       180       240       300       360       420       480       540
```

_5FU

SYMBOL		P	SYMBOL		P	SYMBOL		P
∙∙∙∙∙∙	-1	- -.686	++++++	1.195	- 1.822	■■■■■	3.703	- 4.330
!!!!!!	-.686	- -.059	000000	1.822	- 2.449	■■■■■	4.330	- 4.643
------	-.059	- 0.568	XXXXX	2.449	- 3.076			
======	0.568	- 1.195	888888	3.076	- 3.703			

NOTE: 2363 OBS HIDDEN

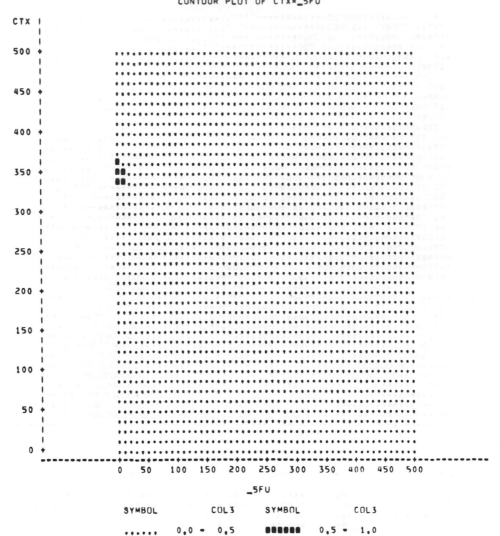

PROPORTIONAL HAZARDS ANALYSIS OF EXPERIMENT 148 - 5FU, CTX

ESTIMATED CONFIDENCE REGION

CONTOUR PLOT OF CTX*_5FU

_5FU

SYMBOL	COL3	SYMBOL	COL3
......	0.0 - 0.5	████████	0.5 - 1.0

NOTE: 511 OBS HIDDEN

PROPORTIONAL HAZARDS ANALYSIS OF EXPERIMENT 148 = 5FU, CTX

Y = RELATIVE HAZARD   MED = MEDIAN

GROUP	X1	X2	Y	MED
1	0	0	1,00000	11,0
2	100	0	0,29619	14,0
3	150	0	0,19163	15,0
4	225	0	0,12379	15,0
5	338	0	0,10460	17,0
6	500	0	0,22951	17,0
7	0	100	0,10381	20,0
8	0	150	0,04432	21,0
9	0	225	0,01758	22,0
10	0	338	0,00969	22,0
11	0	500	0,02198	34,0
12	100	100	0,05120	21,0
13	100	150	0,02821	23,0
14	100	225	0,01640	27,0
15	100	338	0,01609	24,5
16	150	100	0,04274	22,0
17	150	150	0,02675	25,5
18	150	225	0,01883	25,5
19	150	338	0,02464	28,0
20	225	100	0,04047	21,0
21	225	150	0,03067	33,5
22	225	225	0,02876	17,0
23	225	338	0,05797	16,5
24	338	100	0,06085	18,5
25	338	150	0,06150	17,5
26	338	225	0,08885	15,0
27	338	338	0,34340	14,0

PROPORTIONAL HAZARDS ANALYSIS OF EXPERIMENT 148 = 5FU, CTX

Y = RELATIVE HAZARD   MED = MEDIAN

VARIABLE	N	MEAN	STD DEV	MEDIAN	MINIMUM	MAXIMUM
MED	27	20,64814815	5,75261615	21,00000000	11,00000000	34,00000000
Y	27	0,11409066	0,19739527	0,04432366	0,00969285	1,00000000

SPEARMAN CORRELATION COEFFICIENTS / PROB > IRI UNDER H0:RHO=0 / N = 27

	MED	Y
MED	1,00000	=0,85706
MEDIAN OF SURVTIME	0,0000	0,0001
Y	=0,85706	1,00000
	0,0001	0,0000

   The following listing is the second example of the double
precision function subprogram written in Fortran which must be
supplied by the user in order to use the Nelder–Mead optimization procedure. It, JCL to read the data and the data cards
are placed immediately after the Nelder–Mead subroutine in the
card deck. Like the function in the first example, the name is
FN, and it is called by and returns a value to the Nelder–Mead
subroutine. Here, the value of ℓn relative risk is returned.
Data cards required and appropriate JCL are listed in their
correct order.

```
C--------------------------------------------------------------------C
C                                                                    C
C       PROGRAM 'FUNCTION' - CALCULATES VALUE OF FUNCTION TO BE OPTIMIZED   C
C                  (PROPORTIONAL HAZARDS EXAMPLE)                     C
C                                                                    C
C--------------------------------------------------------------------C
C                                                                    C
C                                                                    C
      DOUBLE PRECISION FUNCTION FN(X)
      DOUBLE PRECISION X(4),B(19),CNSTRN(4,2),XPB
      COMMON B,CNSTRN,N
      DO 5 I=1,N
      IF (X(I).LT.CNSTRN(I,1)) GO TO 10
      IF (X(I).GT.CNSTRN(I,2)) GO TO 10
    5 CONTINUE
C                                                                    C
C         CALCULATION OF VALUE OF FUNCTION TO BE OPTIMIZED FOLLOWS    C
C                                                                    C
      FN = B(1)*X(1) + B(2)*X(2) + B(3)*X(1)*X(1) + B(4)*X(2)*X(2) + B(5
     1)*X(1)*X(2)
      RETURN
   10 FN=1.0D38
      RETURN
      END
//GO.SYSIN DD *
```

```
          DATA CARDS ARE PLACED HERE, PUNCHED AS FOLLOWS:


EXP 148 - 5FU, CTX                    PROPORTIONAL HAZARDS PARAMETERS
   800     2     5 .00000001
5FU         0.0        500.
CTX         0.0        500.
       60,        300,
       .01        .01
-.01447346-.026406170.000023060.000037540.00005099
```

The computer output obtained from the Nelder–Mead program using the function given on the preceding page follows. Items output are the same as those discussed in the logistic regression analysis. The optimal dose combination estimated below using the proportional hazards function is 0.0000016 mg/kg of 5-FU and 350.5 mg/kg of CTX.

EXP 148 – 5FU, CTX   PROPORTIONAL HAZARDS PARAMETERS

MAXIMUM NO. ITERATIONS ALLOWED = 800
NO. DRUGS IN THE COMBINATION = 2
CONVERGENCE CRITERION = 0.100D-07

DRUG	REGION CONSTRAINTS		STARTING VALUE	STEP SIZE
5FU	0.0	500.0000	60.0000	0.0100
CTX	0.0	500.0000	300.0000	0.0100

COORDINATES OF INITIAL SIMPLEX		FUNCTION VALUES
60.0100	300.0000	-0.44108D 01
60.0000	300.0100	-0.44108D 01
60.0000	300.0000	-0.44108D 01

175 TRIALS USED

ESTIMATES

PARAMETER	NEXT-TO-BEST	BEST
1	0.1231005D-04	0.1601140D-05
2	0.3505357D 03	0.3505357D 03

FUNCTION VALUES

NEXT-TO-BEST	BEST
-0.4643567D 01	-0.4643567D 01

REFERENCES

1. Olsson, D. M. (1974). A sequential simplex program for
   solving minimization problems. *J. Quality Technology*, *6*,
   53–57.

2. Reinhardt, Patti S. (ed.) (1980). *SAS Supplemental Library
   User's Guide*, SAS Institute, Inc., Cary, North Carolina.

Index

Printed and bound by CPI Group (UK) Ltd, Croydon, CR0 4YY

17/10/2024

01775659-0015